# REPRODUCTIVE PHYSIOLOGY *AND* BIRTH CONTROL

# REPRODUCTIVE PHYSIOLOGY *AND* BIRTH CONTROL

The Writings of
Charles Knowlton and Annie Besant

## S. Chandrasekhar, editor

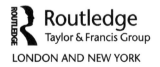

Routledge
Taylor & Francis Group

LONDON AND NEW YORK

Originally published by University of California Press, © 1981 by the Regents of the University of California.

Published 2002 by Transaction Publishers

Published 2017 by Routledge
2 Park Square, Milton Park, Abingdon, Oxon, OX14 4RN
711 Third Avenue, New York, NY 10017, USA

*Routledge is an imprint of the Taylor & Francis Group, an informa business*

Copyright © 2002 by Taylor & Francis.

Library of Congress Catalog Number: 2001057374

Library of Congress Cataloging-in-Publication Data

Chandrasekhar, S. (Sripati), 1918-
 [Dirty filthy book ]
 Reproductive physiology and birth control : the writings of Charles
Knowlton and Annie Besant / S. Chandrasekhar, editor
  p. cm.
 Originally published: "A dirty filthy book". Berkeley : University of California Press, c1981.
 Includes bibliographical references and index.
 ISBN 0-7658-0904-4 (pbk. : alk. paper)
 1. Birth control. 2. Malthusianism. 3. Population policy. 4. Birth control—Religious aspects—Theosophy. 5. Bradlaugh, Charles, 1833-1891. I. Title.

HQ766 .C483 2001
304.6'66—dc21                                              2001057374


ISBN 13: 978-0-7658-0904-9 (pbk)

*I say that this is a dirty, filthy book, and
the test of it is that no human being would allow
that book on his table, no decently educated English
husband would allow even his wife to have it. . . .*

SIR HARDINGE GIFFORD
PROSECUTOR, BRADLAUGH–BESANT TRIAL

TO THE MEMORY OF
ALVIN R. KAUFMAN (1885–1979)
CANADA'S BIRTH CONTROL PIONEER
FOR ALL HIS GENEROUS SUPPORT

# CONTENTS

# PREFACE

In the history of ideas, the fight for both the dissemination and democratization of birth control information constitutes one of the more fascinating and rewarding chapters. And to that chapter, the Charles Bradlaugh–Annie Besant trial (and the role of these two extraordinary British crusaders in the trial as well as in the whole Neo-Malthusian Movement) contributes an exciting and instructive episode.

The court battle and its consequences touched many contemporary issues and personalities. Among the issues were the contents of Charles Knowlton's book that dealt with reproductive physiology (contents that were sometimes ignored and sometimes taken serious notice of by the law on both sides of the Atlantic), its publication with or without pictures ("obscene" or otherwise), and the language and price of the book. The contents, including the author's recommendation of a postcoital douche to prevent conception, pale into insignificance compared to the sex manuals of our contemporary, permissive society. It is difficult for us even to imagine today that the subjects of reproductive physiology, coitus, and conception control were almost literally unmentionable a century ago. As for language, had Dr. Knowlton employed the learned, obscure, and clinical language of his day, his publication might have gone unnoticed by the law and been read only by a handful of medical students and physicians. And last, the price of the book—had it been published at a guinea a copy, thus restricting the sales to a very small minority of the wealthy, the law would not have interfered and the rich alone would have had access to the forbidden knowledge. But the sale of a birth control manual at sixpence, and its clarity and simplicity, made all the difference. The working classes, particularly poor wives, could be informed about and emancipated from unwanted pregnancies. Thus the trial brought out what purported to be the legal obstacles, not only to the dissemination of contraceptive information, but also to its democratization.

As for personalities, the pious public wondered if a cause championed by agnostics and atheists could truly be moral. But, then, apparently most good and worthy causes seemed to be increasingly championed by freethinkers. (Though among the freethinkers and secularists were some radicals who believed only in the demolishment of God and religion and not in the betterment of the lives of the poor.) The conventional and the church-going were somehow always with the establishment and for the status quo.

Then there was the fame—or notoriety, depending on one's point of view—of the two radicals who fought the issue. The British Victorian middle classes were puzzled. They could understand an iconoclast like Charles Bradlaugh, but how could Mrs. Annie Besant, a respectable British woman, talk of sex, and worse, of preventing the divinely ordained consequences of the unmentionable act? These doubts were eagerly fanned by the fundamentalist clergy, with their holier-than-thou attitude toward the whole "scandal" of free thought, secularism, and the birth control movement.

But mild winds of change were blowing across nineteenth-century England. The growth of factories and the gradual industrialization of the country, with all their inherent abuses, had become realities. A scientific outlook was slowly permeating the atmosphere, and restive working classes were in search of both secularism and social welfare. Thus a variety of facts and forces lent support to the cause of birth control and Neo-Malthusianism, and the trial has thus come to constitute a landmark in British social history.

*   *   *

I have been interested in population problems and family planning both as a demographer and later as a public figure in India concerned with the pressures exerted by India's population growth. As one involved in the fight to put family planning on the map of India as an important method of mitigating the incredible poverty of a great majority of India's people, I have been a student of the history of the birth control movement in many lands, knowing that we in India could profit from their successes and failures in promoting family planning as an integral part of the nation's development policies.

As for the two towering personalities of the trial, I had the opportunity of hearing Mrs. Besant speak when, as a small boy, I was taken by my father to hear her address the Theosophical Lodge at Vellore, a town south of Madras City. Mrs. Besant was very much involved with India and its politics, religion, education, and culture, and was extremely popular with audiences throughout India. The hall was packed to overflowing with an admiring audience of several hundred people. Dressed in a sari, she looked to me like a very old woman. But I was overwhelmed with her volley of words and the dominating presence of her personality. As I recall, I did not understand a word of what she said, but I returned home with the impression of having seen and heard a most extraordinary individual.

After I was appointed Lucie Stern Trustee Professor of Sociology at Mills College, Oakland, California, in 1979, I had the opportunity to deliver a series of lectures on world population problems. As a result of student interest, I devoted some attention in that series to the now-forgotten, bitter fight for the freedom to disseminate birth control information and the consequent, gradual biological liberation of women. This book is a partial product of these lectures. Since it is addressed to laymen and university students, as well as to demographers and other social scientists, I have appended some brief notes on names and subjects that may be unfamiliar.

I am indebted to Professors William Petersen, John Dillon, and Stanley Wolpert, and to Grant Barnes and Dan Dixon of the University of California Press for their valuable suggestions. And, as always, I am grateful to my wife for her editorial and secretarial help.

S. Chandrasekhar
Berkeley, California
October 1979

# Introduction

The famous Bradlaugh–Besant trial of 1877–1878 was the culmination of a long and difficult battle fought in London over the freedom to publish Neo-Malthusian birth control material. The Neo-Malthusian issue, more strictly the right to publish a plea for birth control and to disseminate contraceptive information, arose in January 1877, when Charles Watts (1836–1906), a London publisher, pleaded guilty to publishing the American birth control book *Fruits of Philosophy: The Private Companion of Young Married People* by Dr. Charles Knowlton (1800–1850), a Massachusetts physician. This slim volume had been on the list of James Watson (1799–1874), the British publisher, since 1834 (the book was first published in Massachusetts in 1832) and had been sold for him by the Holyoake brothers.[1] But with the death of Watson in 1874, Watts bought the printing plates from Watson's widow and republished the book.

In 1876 Henry Cook, a Bristol bookkeeper, published the same book, interleaved with some illustrations alleged to be obscene, and was arrested and sentenced to two-years hard labor. Watts was not particularly anxious to associate himself with this part of his publishing legacy; but on the advice of Charles Bradlaugh (1833–1891), the redoubtable British freethinker, and his associate on the subject of free thought and secularism, Mrs. Annie Besant (1847–1933), Watts went to Bristol to declare himself the original publisher. Watts was arrested in London and arraigned before the Magistrate in Guildhall.

Thereupon Bradlaugh and Besant published the work, *Fruits of Philosophy*, in the original format but with a new introduc-

1. George Holyoake (1817–1906) and Austin Holyoake (1826–1874) operated a freethought publishing house in London, Messrs. Holyoake and Company.

tion, and informed the police that they planned to sell the book at a particular place and time. They were prosecuted and found guilty, but Bradlaugh found a loophole in the conviction and had the sentence quashed in February 1878.

But we are anticipating our story, for the Bradlaugh–Besant legal battle can be best appreciated against the background of man's long and universal quest for methods of controlling conception.

## MALTHUS AND THE RISE OF NEO-MALTHUSIANISM

*1*

While many thinkers and religious leaders prescribed various ways to increase or maintain the populations of particular cults, groups, tribes, or nations, no one expressed any alarm about the *growth* of population until in 1798 the thirty-two-year-old English clergyman Thomas Robert Malthus anonymously published his long, clearly written, and pessimistic pamphlet, *An Essay on the Principle of Population* with the subtitle *As It Affects the Future Improvement of Society, with Remarks on the Speculation of Mr. Godwin, M. Condorcet and other writers.* With the publication of the first British census in 1801, Malthus enlarged the pamphlet into a full-sized book and in 1803 published it with a changed emphasis and a new subtitle: *A View of Its Past and Present Effects on Human Happiness with an Inquiry into our Prospects Respecting the Future Removal or Mitigation of the Evils which it Occasions.*

The pamphlet, begun as a tract to inveigh against the baseless utopian ideals of certain contemporary writers, had grown into a full-scale study on the population problem. It appeared in various revised and enlarged editions, the sixth and last appearing in 1826, eight years before the death of Malthus.[2] For more than a quarter-century, in fact, his book influenced most discussions of

2. Malthus's *Essay* went into six editions during his lifetime, in 1798, 1803, 1806, 1807, 1817, and 1826. The second and subsequent editions were so full of new data and qualifications that, compared to the first edition, they may well be considered a new book.

demographics. His views continued to be debated for years after his death; they still are today.

Malthus was not without his immediate predecessors on both sides of the Atlantic. In 1751 Benjamin Franklin, the American statesman, brought out his *Observations Concerning the Increase of Mankind and the Peopling of Countries.*[3] Franklin predicted the doubling of the population of the American colonies every twenty years, a prospect that apparently pleased the author. Malthus's English predecessor was Robert Wallace (1697–1771), the Scottish minister and writer on population, who in 1761 published *Various Prospects of Mankind, Nature and Providence.* Wallace was less optimistic than Franklin, for he conjured population growth as a possible obstacle to the socialist millennium in which he believed, but he considered the danger distant and hypothetical.

Thus the problem of population growth was the subject of concern—slight at first but growing with time—in more than one country. No long period passed in any thoughtful society without someone raising the question of human numbers, often of their alarming, burgeoning growth, and occasionally of the threat of their decline and the possibility of eventual depopulation.

*2*

Thomas Robert Malthus, the second son of Daniel Malthus, an Oxford-educated barrister in comfortable circumstances, was born at the Rookery, near Dorking, Surrey, England, on 14 February 1766.[4] He was one of a family of eight children (which number was not considered excessive), having an elder brother and six sisters. Since their father had his own ideas of education, neither Thomas nor his brother went to a public school. Thomas

---

3. Robert Detweiler, "An Observation on the Demographic Theories of Benjamin Franklin," *Population Review,* 19, nos. 1 and 2 (Jan.-Dec. 1975), 41–45.

4. For a brief and incisive review of Malthus's life and views, see William Petersen "Malthusian Theory: A Commentary and Critique," *Population Review,* 5, no. 2 (July 1961).

was educated first by his father and later at a private school in Bath run by a friend of his father, one Richard Graves; later he was a pupil of Gilbert Wakefield, who like Robert's father was a disciple of Rousseau.

In the winter term of 1784, eighteen-year-old Robert Malthus entered Jesus College, Cambridge. He won prizes for his proficiency in both Latin and English Declamation. At Cambridge he majored in mathematics, not in theology as is popularly supposed. In 1788, in his twenty-second year, he graduated as ninth Wrangler, the only Jesus man among the Wranglers of that year.

In 1788 Malthus took orders. In 1791 he obtained his masters degree, and in 1793, at the comparatively early age of twenty-seven, he was admitted to a Fellowship of his college. In 1796 Malthus accepted a curacy at Albury, his father's residence. Here young Malthus wrote his first literary work, a pamphlet attacking Pitt's administration. The pamphlet, we learn, "was well done" (according to Bishop William Otter, a contemporary) but found no publisher and never saw the light of day. When he brought out his *Essay on the Principle of Population* in 1798, the book created such a stir that the first edition was quickly sold out. But if it brought him well deserved fame, it also brought him undeserved abuse.

Malthus continued to reside at the college rather irregularly until 1804, when he resigned his Fellowship on the occasion of his marriage to Harriet Eckersall. In the same year he was appointed Professor of History and Political Economy in the newly founded East India College at Haileybury. The college was not a regular academic center leading to degrees; its purpose was to give general education and training in Indian languages to the civil servants of the East India Company before they sailed to India. (Incidentally, his was the first professorship of political economy established in Britain.)

Malthus, from all accounts, was fortunate in his home life. Mrs. Malthus was evidently a remarkable woman. She was well known as a charming hostess, for "the tradition of Mrs. Malthus's delightful evening parties, at which the elite of the London scientific world were often present, lingered at Haileybury as long as the College lived."[5]

With the publication of the second edition of his book, Malthus finally secured his reputation. During his lifetime he enjoyed the esteem and friendship of many great contemporaries, particularly David Ricardo, with whom he carried on a lengthy correspondence on the economic questions of the day. From 1799 to 1802 he traveled rather extensively in Europe, including Russia, with a view to collecting more data to support his thesis on population and food supply.

Malthus had three children, two sons and a daughter. The youngest, Lucy, died in 1825, when she was only seventeen years old. While this sad break in the family occasioned considerable sorrow, Malthus bore the loss with his usual resignation: "but for the sake of Mrs. Malthus, who felt her loss most acutely, and in the hope of bringing more composure to all their minds, he made a tour upon the Continent with his family, but returned in the Autumn to his ordinary duties at Haileybury and his usual domestic habits."[6]

Malthus wrote other works, some of which deserve to be remembered, though they were all eclipsed by his earliest effort: *The Principles of Political Economy Considered with a View to their Practical Application* (1820), *A Series of Short Studies Dealing with the Corn Laws* (1814–1815), *On Rent* (1815), *The Poor Law* (1817), and *Definitions in Political Economy* (1827). He restated his doctrine of population in an article in the Supplement to the *Encyclopaedia Britannica* (1824) as "A Summary View of the Principle of Population." This was his final statement on the question and it did not differ materially from the view expressed in his *Essay*.

Malthus was elected a Fellow of the Royal Society in 1819,

---

5. *Memorials of Old Haileybury College* (p. 199) as quoted in G. F. McCleary, *The Malthusian Population Theory* (London: Faber and Faber, 1953), p. 169.

6. W. Otter, *Memoir of Robert Malthus* (1836), p. xxxviii.

and later a member of the Institute of France and the Royal Academy of Berlin. He was one of the founders of the Political Economy Club in 1821 and the Royal Statistical Society in 1824.

Malthus and his family spent the Christmas of 1834 at the home of his father-in-law at Claverton, Bath, where a few days later, on 29 December, he died of a heart attack at the age of sixty-eight. He was buried in Bath Abbey and the site is commemorated by a tablet commissioned by Bishop Otter, Malthus's lifelong friend and his contemporary at Cambridge. Harriet Malthus, eleven years younger than her husband, later remarried and survived him by thirty years. Malthus was also survived by his two sons.

## 3

In 1793, when Malthus was twenty-seven, Antoine-Nicolas de Condorcet (1743–1794), the French humanist, mathematician, and philosopher of Voltaire's (1694–1778) circle, secreted himself from Robespierre's secret police in the Paris home of a Madame Vernet. There he wrote his *Esquisse* in six months, all the time sought by the French Revolutionary Tribunal for execution. Though he was influential and was in fact an early revolutionary, he had incurred the displeasure of the party by voting against the execution of the French king and for the abolition of the death penalty itself. The book finished, Condorcet disguised himself, left his hiding place, and managed to escape from Paris; but he was recognized, caught, and imprisoned. He died in detention (committing suicide, according to some accounts) before he could be hanged or guillotined. His book, however, was published in Paris in 1794. In that remarkable book, Condorcet reviews the history of mankind and claims to have found "a natural order in social phenomena making effectively for the continuous improvement of human life."[7] He prophesies the eventual arrival of the millennium, when "racial and national animosities, and inequalities of sex, wealth, education and op-

7. G. F. McCleary, p. 16.

portunity, will disappear; law and institutions will constantly tend to identify individual and collective interests, a universal language will be established; the fruitfulness of the earth will be increased and food obtained from the synthesis of elements and the conquest of disease will be achieved."[8] He concludes: "We have witnessed the development of a new doctrine which is to deliver the final blow to the already tottering structure of prejudice. It is the idea of the limitless perfectibility of the human species."

Although Condorcet's *Esquisse* was published in England in 1795, the coming of the utopia had already been foretold there by William Godwin, poet Shelley's father-in-law, whose *Enquiry Concerning Political Justice* was published in 1793. Godwin predicts the dawn of a society where economic and social equality would be established and where the manual labor of a half-hour would provide the necessities of life to the entire community. According to Godwin, in that society, "There will be no war, no crimes, no administration of justice, as it is called, and no Government. Besides this, there will be neither disease, anguish, melancholy, nor resentment. Every man will seek with ineffable ardour the good of all."[9]

Godwin's *Political Justice* (and the *Enquirer* published in 1797), like Condorcet's *Esquisse*, was inspired by the French Revolution. Among those who believed in the possibility of this utopia was Daniel Malthus, father of Thomas Robert, an English barrister who did not practise but lived in ease as a country squire interested in good causes. He could count among his friends two celebrated men of his times—David Hume and Jean-Jacques Rousseau. Daniel Malthus, who believed ardently in man's eventual attainment of utopia, commended Godwin's book to his thirty-one-year-old son, then a curate at Albury, where his father lived. But the son belonged to a different school. He did not believe in the wishful thinking that promised a utopia of social and economic equality. He told his father that man's

8. Ibid.
9. As quoted in G. F. McCleary, p. 9.

power to produce population was greater than his power to produce subsistence for this population, and that the disparity was decisive enough to militate against the possibility of a utopian society. Thus father and son disputed on the possibility, or rather the impossibility, of man's perfectibility and, indeed, on his ultimate immortality here on earth. As Sir Alexander Gray puts it, "The father and son disputed and the dispute being ended or suspended, young Malthus, moved by the *esprit d'escalier,* proceeded to commit to paper the arguments which would most effectively have cornered his father, had he thought of them in time."[10] This was how Malthus's *Essay on Population* came to be written.

## 4

What did Malthus write?[11] What is the Malthusian population theory? Malthus bases his principles on two postulates: "First, that food is necessary to the existence of man. Secondly, that the passion between the sexes is necessary, and will remain in its present state."[12] Malthus does not elaborate these postulates at length, for they appear to him to be self-evident. He points out that no one could seriously suppose that man could some day live without food. As to the second postulate, he assumes that passion between the sexes is necessary to propagate and perpetuate the species. He does not think that "passion" is diminishing, though man has "progressed" from savagery to civilization; if anything, "passion between the sexes" is being accentuated by the mores of civilization. There is no question of passion ever becoming extinct.

10. Alexander Gray, *The Development of Economic Doctrine* (London: Longmans, 1931), p. 156.

11. For an excellent and detailed study of Malthus and his life and views, see William Petersen, *Malthus* (Cambridge, Mass.: Harvard University Press, 1979).

12. Malthus's *Essay,* 1st ed., p. 11.

Assuming these two postulates to be granted, Malthus lays down the following propositions:

"The power of population is indefinitely greater than the power in the earth to produce subsistence for man.

"Population, when unchecked, increases in a geometrical ratio. Subsistence increases only in an arithmetical ratio. . . ."[13]

The first proposition, that population tends to multiply faster than the means available for its sustenance, is apparently true; and yet it has been a bone of contention ever since man began to think about this particular problem. Malthus was, however, the first to formulate it in this manner. The possible answer that science will be able to increase the means of subsistence or that man will have enough sense to restrain the inordinate growth of population simply evades the question. But it is obvious that population cannot really overrun the means of subsistence, for without subsistence population is bound to perish. The lack of subsistence brings into existence certain undesirable forces that will keep the population in check. As Kingsley Davis rightly points out, "The very fact that numbers are increasing indicates that the means to support them is increasing too. Otherwise mortality would have risen and the population would never have grown to its present size. To think of the world's population as "outrunning" its normal food supply is like thinking of the hind feet of the horse outrunning the front feet."[14]

The second proposition, concerning the geometrical and arithmetical ratios, is impressive but unsound. The growth of population is represented by a geometrical increase: 1, 2, 4, 8, 16, 32, 64, 128, 256; and the increase of the means of subsistence is represented by arithmetical progression: 1, 2, 3, 4, 5, 6, 7, 8, 9. Each term corresponds to a period of twenty-five years, and a glance at the figures shows that if unchecked population should double every twenty-five years, while subsistence merely in-

13. Malthus, *Essay*, pp. 13–14.
14. Kingsley Davis, *Human Society* (New York: Macmillan, 1949), p. 612.

creases by an equal amount during each of these periods. The divergence between the two series grows with alarming rapidity. In the example above, the population has grown to twenty-seven times the means of subsistence in 225 years.

These "revolting ratios" loom large in all Malthusian controversies. Though they are true of the lives of most organisms, they cannot be taken as an exact measure of human reproduction. The ratios are at best a vivid way of saying that man tends to multiply beyond his means of subsistence. Malthus points out that "The germs of existence contained in this earth, if they could freely develop themselves, would fill millions of worlds in the course of a few thousand years. Necessity, that imperious, all pervading law of Nature, restrains them within the prescribed bounds. The race of plants and the race of animals shrink under this great restrictive law; and man cannot by any efforts of reason escape from it."[15]

Since "population can never actually increase beyond the lowest nourishment capable of supporting it," some checks to population must be constantly in operation. And these checks are positive and preventive. The positive checks are those influences that increase the death rate, "the whole train of epidemics, wars, plagues and famines." The preventive checks are those influences that lead to a diminution of the birth rate, such as postponement of marriage and moral restraint.

Malthus himself has summarized for us his population theory in three celebrated propositions:

1. Population is necessarily limited by the means of subsistence.

2. Population invariably increases when the means of subsistence increases, unless prevented by some powerful and obvious check.

3. These checks, and the checks that repress the superior power of population and keep its effects on a level with the means of subsistence, are all resolvable by either moral restraint or vice and misery.

15. Malthus, *Essay,* 2nd ed., p. 6.

## 5

Was Malthus right? How relevant is his population theory today? Before these two questions are answered, some misconceptions about Malthus and his views need correcting. It is commonly supposed that Malthus advocated contraception. Sometimes it is held that Malthus *would* have advocated contraception had he known about it. In fact, contraception is very much older than Malthus, and he certainly knew about it. But he *never* advocated contraception; on the contrary, he indirectly condemned it.[16] Promoters of modern birth control need not, therefore, necessarily label themselves "Malthusians."

Another popular mistake about Malthus is that he was a "gloomy prophet," a person who foretold the dire consequences of an excessive multiplication of the human population. Malthus did not forecast doom in the distant future. He simply said that man's power to produce population is so much greater than his power to produce subsistence that it leads to vice and misery—not in the distant future but here and now, as it always has. Nor did Malthus recommend war, disease, and famine as solutions to the problems of overpopulation. These and other misrepresentations of the Malthusian doctrine can be explained in general by a peculiar human trait: when a man's ideas become famous, everybody talks about them and criticizes them, but few read them. The misunderstanding of one's admirers, even one's followers, is often the price of fame. Everybody was out to hail, attack, or refute Malthus, but few bothered to study his essay with its numerous qualifications and modifications.

Was Malthus right? The Malthusian "principle" was basically correct in its application to the effect of population on subsistence, not only in Malthus's native Britain but also in many

---

16. Regarding birth control, Malthus asserted, "I should always particularly reprobate any artificial and unnatural modes of checking population, both on account of their immorality and their tendency to remove a necessary stimulus to industry. If it were possible for each married couple to limit by a wish the number of their children, there is certainly reason to fear that the indolence of the human race would be very greatly increased." Malthus, *Essay,* 6th ed., 1826, p. 543.

European countries that he had visited and studied. The principle of population was sound as a piece of deductive and, in later editions, inductive logic. And while the conditions he deplored in England and Europe have been mitigated by innovations Malthus could not anticipate, his principle still holds true in many underdeveloped countries of the modern world, where these innovations have either not taken firm root or have not yet been implemented.

Since the days of Malthus, four factors have relieved the pressure of population against the means of subsistence or even resources in the West. First, there was the large-scale emigration to the new world. Second, Europe witnessed a tremendous increase in both agricultural and industrial production. The law of diminishing returns in agriculture has been more than offset by the law of increasing returns in industry. Third, and perhaps the most important of all, is the spread of contraception and the consequent decline in the birth rate. And last is the relative emancipation of women. Malthus could not foresee the changes in the economic condition and the mental attitude of women that have caused them to marry later in life, as well as to have fewer children after marriage. In fact, one can read the *Essay* from cover to cover without encountering a passage that indicates Malthus ever thought women had anything to do with population.

Malthus assumed that only misery and suffering and the fear of more suffering could compel the underprivileged to control their birth rate. If this were true, India's masses would have reduced their fertility long ago. The population problems of the third world contradict this assumption of Malthus. However, it would hardly be fair to attack Malthus for erroneous reasoning on the ground that he failed to foresee the unfolding of all these factors that appear to falsify some of his propositions.

There is another line of attack on Malthus, that of the Marxists. When Malthus maintained that the poor were responsible for their poverty, that a way out of their condition was through celibacy and continence, he thought he was furthering the interests of the poor laborer. In effect, it was criminal for pauper boys and girls to marry and beget large numbers of children whom they could not support and who eventually became a burden on the taxpayer. In this he was supported by the leading economist of the day, Nassau Senior, Professor of Political Economy at Oxford, who wrote to Malthus in 1829: "We have the poor laws to increase our numbers." But when the Malthusian principle was interpreted to mean a denial of poor relief and a refusal to encourage contraception as a means of population control (the difficulties of Malthus, a clergyman, on this question must be appreciated), Malthus appeared inhuman and utterly unsympathetic to the wretched plight of the needy. But if poverty is to be explained in terms of teeming numbers and the pressure population exerts on resources, then the very basis of Marxism is undermined. Marxism, in a word, explains poverty as a result of the exploitation of workers by the existing capitalistic economic order. Hence the Marxian attack on Malthusianism.

In a real sense, Malthus did prove to be against progressive thinking. His inquiry into the social condition of the Britian of his day did not lead him to conclude that something had to be done or could be done to mitigate the misery of the underprivileged. In fact the *Essay*, with ingenious arguments, demonstrates the author's firm belief in the status quo and contains a latent plea for not doing anything to effect change. To him poverty and low levels of living were inevitable, and social reforms designed to alleviate the miserable conditions of the working classes only increased their plight. One may reasonably conclude that the major objective of Malthus's thesis was to discredit Condorcet's belief that disease, poverty, and war are eradicable evils.

The innovation of modern contraception has taken the sting out of the Malthusian principle. As Professor David Glass rightly points out, "Last of all, this very spread of family limitation has itself destroyed an important part of Malthus's argument. Birth control may, in Malthus's terms, constitute a vice, though it is certainly not regarded as such by millions of married couples. But at least the ability easily to limit one's family has not, as Malthus feared, reduced individuals to indolence or society to stagnation. On the contrary, it has been one of the ways through which new incentives and aspirations have been able to work with effect. Whatever the validity of the Malthusian theory, Malthus's precepts of conduct have lost their relevance as a means of preventing a conflict between population and resources."[17]

Today, more than ever, the population problems of the world have become insistent, bringing Malthus to the fore again. At some stage of all demographic discussions, we go back to Malthus, our *pradhāna achārya* (first serious teacher) on this subject.

Although Malthus, the clergyman and economist, was concerned about the poverty of the British working class and talked of the predicament of population growth and the want of resources to support the population, he ignored and evaded birth control as an effective solution. Malthus pleaded for moral restraint instead. Charles Knowlton, an obscure American physician on the other side of the Atlantic, gave thought to the same problem. He saw only too clearly the financial dilemma of young married couples and proposed a relatively easy solution: birth control.

Knowlton was born in 1800, two years after the publication of the first edition of Malthus's *Essay on the Principle of Population*. And Malthus died in 1834, two years after the first edition of Knowlton's tract *The Fruits of Philosophy* was published and before it reached Britain. But even before Knowlton, an uneducated London tailor, Francis Place, concerned about the problem, recommended contraception instead of moral restraint to the British working classes.

### FRANCIS PLACE AND THE "DIABOLICAL HAND BILLS"

Judging from the available literature, especially pamphlets of the period, many thoughtful writers seem to have reflected on the human condition of nineteenth-century England, particularly the population numbers and their relation to poverty, hun-

17. D. V. Glass, ed., *Introduction to Malthus* (London: Watts, 1953), pp. 49–50.

ger, and squalor among the working classes. These writers had been looking for some feasible answer (within the straitjacket of the establishment's puritanical attitude toward sex and morals) to the problem of effectively divorcing the sex act from its natural consequence—children. The dilemma of the sexual enjoyment one wanted and the burden of children one did not want could not be resolved. The difficulties were numerous, ranging all the way from ignorance of basic human reproductive physiology to religious obscurantism on the sex question and the total hypocritical cultural milieu of mid-Victorian prudery. Until Francis Place, a hard-working, thoughtful London tailor, became the first English advocate and propagandist of birth control, in the modern sense of the term, no one even dared to think aloud publicly that some kind of a mechanical barrier used by the female before coitus might possibly be an answer.

Place, "the radical breeches-maker of Charing Cross," was born on November 3, 1771, to an uneducated, poverty-stricken bailiff who maintained a debtors' prison in London. Place had a miserable home life and received no schooling worth the name. When he was thirteen years old he was apprenticed to a breeches maker with whom he worked hard for the next four years to learn tailoring. At seventeen he became a journeyman (a worker learning a trade and working for another person). When not yet twenty he married sixteen-year-old Elizabeth Chadd, "a fine handsome young woman, tall, well grown and womanish in her appearance." They lived in one room of a court off the Strand and, since their combined wages hardly made ends meet, they lived in genteel but grinding poverty.

Within two years of Place's marriage, the breech makers struck for higher wages; after a three-month struggle the strike failed. While the workers returned to work on the employers' terms and at their original wages, Place, a strike leader and organizer of the trade club (the precursor of the trade and labor unions), was refused reinstatement. For the next six months the young couple faced extreme privation that bordered on starvation. During this period they saw their child die of smallpox. But Place's physical and mental fortitude was such that during his forced idleness he studied laboriously works dealing with economics, history, law, and mathematics and largely made up for his lack of formal education.

In 1794 he became secretary of his trade club and later secretary for several other similar organizations of carpenters, plumbers, and other artificers. In the same year he joined the London Corresponding Society, the labor section of the democratic movement of the time. The Society's demands included manhood suffrage, annual parliaments, and salaries for Members of Parliament. Since he was able and businesslike, Place usually became the chairman at their meetings.

In 1799 he began to concentrate on his personal trade and financial affairs. By dint of hard work, he was able to build up his own business and in partnership with a fellow worker soon opened a tailor's shop on Charing Cross. Though within two years the partnership broke up, Place bought the business and moved into his own shop nearby. He became a success and transformed himself from "an underfed journeyman into a prosperous tradesman." By 1816 Place made enough profits to hand over his business to his eldest son and retire.

From that time he was able to devote himself to study and politics and spend more time with his books in the precious library he had built behind his tailoring shop. There, unknown to his customers, his friends—politicians and publicists—met and discussed the politics of the day. In 1807 he took a leading part in the general elections, campaigning for Sir Francis Burdett, an independent candidate for Westminster. He began writing for the newspapers and for working-class organs and came to be widely known to politicians and political thinkers. He enjoyed the friendship of such distinguished men as William Godwin (1756–1836), James Mill (1773–1836), Jeremy Bentham (1784–1832), Robert Owen (1771–1858), and others.

After a decade of gathering facts and figures, preparing petitions and memoranda, helping Members of Parliament and other politicians with valuable general economic and social data, and working behind the scenes, he achieved his greatest success

in getting the laws against Combinations (trade unions) repealed. In 1825 he successfully prevented their reinstatement.
He thus laid securely the foundations of British Trade Unionism.
He also supported the Reform Bill of 1832 and drafted the Peoples' Charter in 1838 (from which the Chartists derived their
name) for the London Workingmen's Association. In short he
became a political gadfly in the English radical politics of
the day.

But of all his activities, his work as a Neo-Malthusian propagandist, pleading for and disseminating birth control information to working-class couples, is to us most noteworthy. As a self-
educated man from the slums, Place knew firsthand how a large
family was a major barrier to the economic well-being of the
working class. It was Place who was responsible for preparing,
printing, and distributing leaflets or hand bills entitled "To the
Married of Both Sexes." The objective of these leaflets was to
explain in simple language how a workingman and his wife
could prevent conception and avoid a large family.

"Large families," said the leaflet, "led to poverty. Yet the
means of prevention were simple and harmless. The method
which seemed most likely to succeed in this country, since it depended on the female, consisted in 'a piece of sponge about an
inch square, being placed in the vagina previous to coition, and
afterwards withdrawn by means of a double twisted thread, or
bobbin, attached to it'."[18] According to the leaflet there would
be no harmful consequences, nor would sexual enjoyment be diminished.

There were two other hand bills addressed "To the Married of
Both Sexes in Genteel Life" and "To the Married of Both Sexes
of the Working People." The working-class recipients of the leaflet were told simply and truthfully, "You cannot fail to see that
this address is intended solely for your good. It is quite impossi-

18. Peter Fryer, *The Birth Controllers* (London: Corgi Books, 1967), p.
43. For a delightful survey of birth control through the ages, this book is
recommended. The present writer has drawn some material for this essay
from it.

ble that those who address you can receive any benefit from it, beyond the satisfaction which every benevolent person, every true Christian, must feel at seeing you comfortable, healthy and happy."[19]

Place's only published work deals with neither the Combination Laws, the Chartist demands, nor the Reform Bill, but with the population question. It is entitled *Illustrations and Proofs of the Principle of Population* (published in 1822) and contains some of his best work. It replied to Godwin's *Enquirer* (1797). More than a century later, Norman E. Himes, the American sociologist chronicler of contraceptive methods, reprinted this book with the subtitle "Being the First Work on Population in the English Language Recommending Birth Control, now Exactly Reproduced with an Introduction Demonstrating Francis Place as the Founder of the Modern Birth Control Movement."[20]

In addition to this book and the hand bills, Place carried on Neo-Malthusian propaganda for more than twenty years, through conversation, correspondence, and brief pieces in working-class papers. While the book was not much of a success, for it sold only an estimated five hundred copies, the hand bills reached a wide working-class readership between London and Manchester.

To Place, dedicated as he was to the promotion of the welfare of the working classes, the population question loomed large. To him the Malthusian recommendation of moral restraint to working-class couples was nothing short of an absurdity. As James Field points out, "His [Place's] own early marriage had been his salvation. He had failed to live decently in celibacy even to the age of nineteen; and, for the man of the laboring class who awaited assured means of supporting a family before taking a wife, the horror of this youthful experience foretold to him hope-

19. Peter Fryer, p. 47. Copies of these leaflets are mounted in the British Museum's Place Collection.
20. George Allen and Unwin, London; and Houghton Mifflin Co., Boston and New York.

less immorality. But experience no less emphatically warned him that early marriage meant many children."[21]

Place crystallized the latent longings of men and women into a social movement that had as its sole commitment separating the sexual appetite from the desire for progeny. Man had endeavoured from time immemorial to divorce the sex act from its natural consequences by a simple, effective, and harmless method, but did not know how. In the English-speaking world, Place was the first to bring to the public notice an effective answer through his "diabolical" but God-sent hand bills.

Once the ice was broken, the dissemination of birth control information began to move relatively fast. Place in a way influenced Richard Carlile (1790–1843), freethinker and Neo-Malthusian, publishing his daring, "indelicate" *Every Woman's Book* or *What is Love* (1825). Robert Dale Owen (1801–1877), the American reformer and eldest son of Robert Owen, wealthy Scottish manufacturer and philanthropist and Utopian socialist who founded the Utopian community of New Lanark near Manchester, England, brought a copy of *Every Woman's Book* to the United States on a brief visit in 1827. Finding that Carlile's book was being secretly circulated and read, and that an edition was even being pirated in his name, Owen felt compelled to write his own book on the subject. In 1831 be brought out in the United States his *Moral Physiology; or, A Brief and Plain Treatise on the Population Question.* Owen recommended *coitus interruptus* (a method widely known and used) and therefore cannot claim to have pioneered the advocacy of contraception in the modern sense. But his work, as well as Place's hand bills, influenced Charles Knowlton to write his *Fruits of Philosophy*, the *corpus delicti* of the Bradlaugh–Besant trial. It can therefore be argued that Place's work set in motion a chain reaction that led to the landmark trial.

To come back to Place's personal life. After a happy marriage of thirty-six years, he lost his wife to cancer in 1827. In 1830 he

21. James A. Field, "The Early Propagandist Movement in English Population Theory," *Bulletin* of the American Economic Association (1911), p. 220.

remarried and this proved to be an unhappy marriage. He died at the end of 1853, in his eighty-third year. Ironically enough, the man who crusaded so strenuously for small families among the British working class fathered fifteen children, five of whom died in infancy.

Today we remember Francis Place not so much for what he wrote as for what he did in recommending birth control to the poor and the needy with compassion, sympathy, and hope—attributes characteristic of all his activities.

## The Life and Work of Knowlton
### and His FRUITS OF PHILOSOPHY

Charles Knowlton was born in Templeton, Worcester County, Massachusetts, on May 10, 1800. The son of Stephen and Comfort White Knowlton, he was descended from English forebears who emigrated to America in the seventeenth century. Knowlton studied medicine and became a qualified physician. He was, however, almost entirely self-taught, a phenomenon possible in those days. Before he was twenty-one, he had worked for and studied with several medical practitioners in Massachusetts and New Hampshire. At Winchendon, Massachusetts, Knowlton was befriended by Richard Stuart and his family. Stuart helped cure Knowlton of wet dreams by a series of electric shocks. In 1821 Knowlton married Tabitha Stuart, an attractive seventeen-year-old former schoolmate and the daughter of his benefactor. It was a happy marriage and his wife stood by him during all the major and minor tribulations incidental to the life of a free-thinker and birth control pioneer.

In 1821 Knowlton continued his study of medicine with Dr. Charles Wilder of Templeton. Later he entered the New Hampshire Medical Institute (now Dartmouth Medical School). He was desperately poor, and to pay the tuition at Dartmouth and have a chance to dissect, he "resurrected" a cadaver, for which he spent sixty days in jail and was fined two hundred dollars (paid by his father) towards costs for grave robbing and illegal dissection. He received his M.D. degree from the Medical Department of Dartmouth College in 1824.

During his brief imprisonment, Knowlton devoted his forced leisure in the Worcester County jail to some serious reflection on the human condition. Later, while practicing at Hawley in west Massachusetts, he completed the work begun in the prison on the intellectual phenomenon of man about 1825. Finding no publisher, he printed a thousand copies at his own expense in 1829 but found selling them more difficult than he had anticipated. The title of the book was as formidable as its contents and probably frightened away possible buyers: *Elements of Modern Materialism: Inculcating the Idea of a Future State, in which all will be more happy, under whatever circumstances they may be placed, than if they experienced no misery in this life.* Since he could not sell copies at Hawley, he piled them into a carriage and drove off to New York; unfortunately, the booksellers there would not touch them. On a second trip to New York, he was arrested for peddling his books without a license. He had to sell some of his private effects to pay off the printer. Thus his venture in publishing his first book, which apparently made the first American argument for what is now called Behaviorism, proved an unhappy failure. What Knowlton appeared to say was that almost everything people thought or did was determined in a machine-like manner and that there was no sense of real freedom or deliberate choice. Everything including man was merely the product of chance. This, coupled with some principles of free thought, he explained in a verbose and obscure manner.

In 1831 he set up his medical practice in the small town of Ashfield, Massachusetts. His agnostic views were not popular among the conventional, puritanical, church-going New England residents of the town. But as a physician he was popular, and expectant mothers in Ashland and beyond would rather have Dr. Knowlton than anyone else deliver their babies.

Knowlton had been interested for some years in methods of preventing conception. As a thoughtful man and physician, he had realized that an excessive number of births was not only a financial burden on young couples but also a strain on the health of young mothers. He had, therefore, prepared a slender manuscript on methods of preventing conception, which essay he loaned to those of his patients who asked for such advice. When he discovered that some of them profited by his methods (most of his contemporary physicians were squeamish about popularizing such knowledge), he decided to publish them in book form.

Thus in January 1832 the book, under the harmless title *Fruits of Philosophy: the Private Companion of Young Married People, by a Physician*, was published anonymously in New York and priced at fifty cents a copy.

*Fruits of Philosophy* was the first popularly written medical guide on how to prevent conception in the English language, apart from Place's hand bills, and it was priced within the reach of needy husbands and wives. Although a year earlier, in January 1831, Robert Dale Owen brought out his slim book, *Moral Physiology*, dealing with more or less the same subject, it was more a sociological and economic tract and, as noted above, recommended only one non-clinical method, withdrawal. Knowlton's publication was essentially medical, for which reason, as Norman E. Himes points out, Knowlton may be considered the American founder of contraceptive medicine. For almost a century his book had a considerably greater influence than Owen's book on the sexual behavior of the English-speaking people on both sides of the Atlantic, thanks, among other factors, to the Bradlaugh–Besant trial.

The book not only answers the conventional arguments against birth control but explains its numerous advantages. It "begins by answering the most familiar contemporary arguments against contraception. Such practices, it was said, would lead to illicit intercourse. But a female's chastity, if it could be overcome, could be overcome without the knowledge this book conveyed. It was said also that such practices were against nature. But civilized life was one continued battle against nature. Conception control would prevent overpopulation; mitigate the evil of prostitution by making early marriage possible; reduce poverty, ignorance and crime; help prevent hereditary diseases, and preserve and improve the species; reduce the number of artificial abortions and diminish infanticide; and prevent the ill-health caused to women by excessive childbearing or habitual abortion. The idea of 'spacing,' and its benefits, was inherent in Knowlton's thought."[22]

22. Peter Fryer, pp. 114–115. See also Norman E. Himes, *Medical History of Contraception* (New York: Schocken Books, 1970), passim.

23

What are the merits of Dr. Knowlton's book? It had intrinsic medical value as well as historical importance. As Dr. Himes points out, "*The Fruits of Philosophy* is the most important treatise on birth control technique for seventeen centuries; the greatest since the chapter in Sorano's *Gynecology* (2nd century A.D.). Though we have learned much in the last century, the point of view which Knowlton here expresses is essentially modern. . . . Though Knowlton's physiology needs amendment in the light of more recent advances, the tone and point of view are, on the whole, surprisingly modern."[23]

What Knowlton advocated was chemical methods and douching, using an "astringent vegetable" infusion or soda bicarbonate. "His originality," Himes goes on, "lay in suggesting that the vagina should be syringed two or three times, soon after the male emission, with a liquid which would not merely dislodge nearly all the semen but also destroy the fecundating property of that which remained. There were various liquids that would do this. Most convenient of all was a solution of alum."[24] He added that liberal use of cold water would be a never-failing preventive. Knowlton's physiology of human reproduction needs a lot of updating. But judged by the knowledge of the day, it is surprising that the book does not contain more errors than it does.

While the book was not noticed by the lay press, and while the professional press took a long time, some eleven years, to publish a review in the *Boston Medical and Surgical Journal*, the legal authorities in the notoriously puritanical state of Massachusetts were in some hurry to prevent the information in Knowlton's book from reaching the people. Knowlton had three encounters with the law because of the book. In 1832, the year of publication, he was fined fifty dollars and costs at Taunton, Massachusetts, on the complaint of a local lawyer whose own pamphlet accused Knowlton of making the world's oldest profession easy and devoid of its "inconveniences and dangers." On

23. Norman E. Himes, "Introductory Notice," to *Fruits of Philosophy* by Charles Knowlton (Mount Vernon: Peter Pauper Press, 1927), p. v.
24. Peter Fryer, pp. 115–116.

December 10, 1832, on the complaint of a jealous physician at Cambridge, Massachusetts (the medical profession itself is often the greatest obstacle to medical advancement), he was sentenced, despite his *angina pectoris*, to three months hard labor in the House of Correction at Cambridge (January to March 1833) for distributing his book. In 1834–1835, at Greenfield, Massachusetts, Knowlton was again hauled into court. The prosecutions, originating in this instance with an Ashfield clergyman, resulted in a *nolle prosequi*, the jury having been unable to agree on two previous occasions.

These prosecutions did not stop the sale of the book. It went through nine editions in Knowlton's lifetime. While he suffered much for his authorship, he must certainly have enjoyed his book's popularity. And after his death, thanks to the Bradlaugh–Besant trial, Knowlton became internationally famous and his book an incredible bestseller for some time.

Knowlton was, however, no crusader. His later life was quiet and uneventful. He occasionally promoted the cause of free speech and periodically contributed articles on clinical subjects to medical journals. In 1844 he was elected a Fellow of the Massachusetts Medical Society, an honor he enjoyed until his death. He simply settled down as a good citizen of Ashfield, accepted and respected by the members of the community. Little is known of his family. We know that he had five children, one of whom, Charles Lorenzo Knowlton, practiced medicine at Ashfield and later in Northampton, Massachusetts. We also know of his son-in-law, who abridged Knowlton's autobiography, which appeared in the *Boston Medical and Surgical Journal* in 1851, a year after his death. The account stops in 1829, the year before the publication of *Fruits of Philosophy*, and hence Knowlton's later years have been left undocumented.

## The Bradlaugh–Besant Trial, 1877–1878

Knowlton's *Fruits of Philosophy* triumphantly voyaged across the Atlantic and appeared in England in its first British edition in 1833, issued by James Watson. The subtitle, *The Private Companion of Married People*, was changed to *The Private Companion of Married Couples* in what was apparently the first authorized English edition. Its periodic publication by different publishers in England ran a smooth course for some four decades until it became the subject of the epic trial, Regina v. Charles Bradlaugh and Annie Besant in 1877–1878.[25] During those forty-four years, 1833–1877, 40,000 copies had been sold.

We may briefly recall the circumstances leading to the trial. When in 1877 Charles Watts was prosecuted for the publication of Knowlton's book, Charles Bradlaugh and Annie Besant were filled with "wrath and dismay" that he should be so cowardly as to plead guilty of publishing an "obscene" book. Thereupon, to establish the right to publish contraceptive information, they published the book under the auspices of their own Free Thought Publishing Society. This led to their arrest and trial.

### CHARLES BRADLAUGH, 1833–1891

Charles Bradlaugh, the formidable freethinker, orator, and secularist, was born on September 26, 1833, in one of London's squalid slums. After a scanty and scrappy education, which ended when he was ten, he became an errand boy in the office of his father, who worked as a solicitor's clerk. The boy's early en-

25. *2 Law Reports, Queen's Bench Division,* 569, reversed in *3 Law Reports, Queen's Bench Division,* 607. See also the Special Report of the trial in the High Court of Justice, Queen's Bench Division, June 18, 1877. For an unofficial report of the trial, see *The Queen v. Charles Bradlaugh and Annie Besant* (London: Free Thought Publishing Co., 1878), pp. 3–32.

THE BRADLAUGH-BESANT TRIAL

thusiasm for Christianity subsided after his study of the Thirty-Nine Articles of the Church of England and the four synoptic gospels. After some unsuccessful attempts on the part of his parents and employer at straightening out his heterodox views, Bradlaugh left his home and job and found shelter in the home of Eliza Sharples Carlile, the widow of the well-known free-thinker Richard Carlile. Here he fell in love with Hypatia,[26] the widow's eldest daughter.

He began studying scriptures, law, and various other subjects and addressing audiences; his fame as a fluent and forceful speaker spread. His first pamphlet, *A Few Words on the Christian's Creed* (1850), was written when he was seventeen years old.

Unable to eke out a livelihood by selling coal and later buckskin braces—for his anti-religious views were detrimental to his success as a businessman—he enlisted in the army in 1850 and left it after three years.

His subsequent career was full of incidents that made him a rationalist *par excellence* and a champion of the freedom of the press and other worthy causes. In 1855 he became well known by championing the right of public assembly in Hyde Park. By this time Bradlaugh had become famous as "an iconoclast" and a "powerful and pugnacious lecturer, debater and pamphleteer." He also fought numerous battles championing the right of free speech, the most impressive at Plymouth in 1861.

In 1855 Bradlaugh married Susannah Hooper; they had three children, two daughters and a son. After fifteen years of marriage the Bradlaughs broke up. Mrs. Bradlaugh became an alco-

26. Hypatia was a pagan philosopher of Alexandria who was torn to pieces by Christians in A.D. 415. This woman's name was a favorite for free-thinkers. Carlile and Eliza Sharples named their eldest daughter, born in 1830, after her, and Charles Bradlaugh named his elder daughter after Carlile's.
Whenever Mrs. Besant was complimented on her oratorical ability, "she liked to remark whimsically to her friends, she ought to be a good orator since she had been practising for twelve thousand years, and eloquence was one of her most famous characteristics in her lives as the philosopher Hypatia and the monk Bruno"—Arthur H. Nethercot, *The Last Four Lives of Annie Besant* (Chicago: University of Chicago Press, 1963), p. 167.

holic and Bradlaugh bore the sorrow silently. By 1877 Mrs. Bradlaugh and two children had died, leaving behind the elder daughter, Hypatia, who became Mrs. H. Bradlaugh Bonner, surviving Bradlaugh for many years.

In 1860 Bradlaugh started a magazine, "The National Reformer" (1860–1893), to aid him in his task of disseminating his rationalist ideas and ideals. The magazine's avowed support of Atheism, Republicanism, and Neo-Malthusianism and its scathing attack on the British religious, social, and sexual prejudices of the time were enough to have it classified under the "cheap newspaper" category, in accordance with the provisions of an obsolete law, revived in 1868, purporting to define bounds of decency in the press. Every cheap magazine (according to the revived law) was required to deposit 800 pounds as security against possible blasphemous or seditious libel.

Part of Bradlaugh's political activity through the years had involved attempts to free the press from repressive and hostile legislation of various kinds, and in almost all his encounters with the government in this regard he had been successful. He saw in the revival of this law a further menace to a free press, and so he defied its enforcement. His response to the government's order to stop publishing his paper was to announce in the next issue that it was "Printed in Defiance of Her Majesty's Government." He won the case after two prosecutions, and the law was repealed. This success earned him the praise of John Stuart Mill, who wrote to him: "You have gained a very honourable success in obtaining a repeal of this mischievous Act by your persevering resistance."

Bradlaugh contested the Parliamentary seat from Northampton, but he was defeated twice, in 1868 and again in 1874. Ultimately, after twelve years of tireless campaigning, he won the seat for Northampton in the 1880 general election. But surprisingly the battle was not over, and his fight to take his seat inside Parliament was as remarkable as his struggles outside it had been.

After a long and sensational fight to be seated as a Member of the House of Commons, a fight that involved several exclusions, a re-election, and considerable litigation (because of his desire to make an affirmation and not take an oath), Bradlaugh finally succeeded in taking his seat in January 1886, when the new Speaker of the House of Commons insisted on his being allowed to take the "oath" by affirmation. (An oath calls upon God to witness to the truth of what one says; an affirmation is a solemn declaration made under the penalties of perjury by a person who conscientiously declines taking an oath.) When the long fight was finally over, the public had got used to Bradlaugh; his transparent integrity and sincerity and his contempt for mere popularity gained him increasing respect. His major achievement as a Member of Parliament was the Oaths Amendment Act of 1888 by which freethinkers were permitted the right to affirm in cases when an oath had been required before.

He also supported worthwhile foreign causes, taking an interest in the struggles of Garibaldi, Mazzini, and home rule for Ireland. In 1889 Bradlaugh collapsed from physical exhaustion. He voyaged to distant India to recover his health as well as to address the Indian National Congress in Bombay at its annual session when Sir William Wedderburn presided. Indians who expected fireworks from this radical reformer were said to have been disappointed by his somewhat moderate speech. But throughout his life he so championed the cause of India, both inside and outside the House of Commons and whenever an opportunity arose, that he won the appellation of "Member of Parliament for India." He died in 1891, two years after his return to London.

ANNIE WOOD BESANT, 1847–1933

*1*

Considered one of the most remarkable women of her day, Annie Wood Besant, of three-fourths Irish descent, was born in London on October 1, 1847, a century before India's independence.[27] In her life of some eighty-six years she played, with remarkable dedication and apparent sincerity, many roles, some

27. For an excellent and definitive biography of Annie Besant, see Arthur H. Nethercot's two volumes: *The First Five Lives of Annie Besant* (Chicago: University of Chicago Press, 1960) and *The Last Four Lives of Annie Besant* (Chicago: University of Chicago Press, 1963).

of them contradicting others: she was a devout Christian theologian, an ardent atheist and freethinker, an avowed birth controller and Neo-Malthusian, a Fabian socialist and feminist, a science teacher and trade unionist, an author, editor, publisher, "Indian nationalist," orator, social reformer, and a Theosophist.

Annie was born to Emily Roche Morris and Dr. William Wood, physician, mathematician, and religious sceptic. She was the only daughter of a family of three children. At the age of five she experienced the untimely death of her father from a surgical accident and the subsequent loss of her brother, Alfred.

Wood's death left the family almost destitute and necessitated a move to Harrow. There Mrs. Wood rented a house, renovating it into a boarding house for some of the Harrow boys. It was here that Annie came under the guidance of Miss Ellen Marryat, a good Samaritan and teacher, and the youngest sister of a well-known novelist of the day, who persuaded Mrs. Wood to allow Annie to live with her. For the next five years Annie was brought up by Miss Marryat, in the company of other boys and girls staying in her home. Their private education was progressive for that time. Annie's studies included Latin, German, French, history, geography, theology, and considerable Bible study. Her education with Miss Marryat culminated in travel to Paris and Bonn.

In 1863 Annie returned to her mother. Later, in 1878, she would be one of the first women to attend London University. Thus she was considerably better educated than most women of her day.

Under the religious upbringing of the missionary-minded Miss Marryat, Annie developed a martyr complex: "Once she envisioned herself preaching to a vast crowd and converting them to her new religion; and then, brought back to reality, she regretted that she had been born too late to suffer for her beliefs as the old martyrs had done."[28] According to Nethercot, at an early age, Annie was to dream of herself as a martyr fighting for various unpopular causes.

28. As quoted in Arthur H. Nethercot, *The First Five Lives of Annie Besant*, p. 12.

Later, when she was working at a mission church as a volunteer, she met the Rev. Frank Besant, a conventional and prim young deacon of the church, and married him in 1867. Annie was twenty and husband Frank was twenty-seven years old. As she described it, "out of sheer weakness and fear of inflicting pain I drifted into an engagement with a man I did not pretend to love."[29] She was unhappy in her role and surroundings; after numerous quarrels and separations and the birth of two children, Digby and Mabel, the marriage of six years ended in a legal separation.

Besant later wrote that after marriage she and her husband discovered their profound ignorance of sex. This experience taught her the value of sex education. She had felt that the size of their family should be limited to two children, but her husband did not. They argued bitterly, fought over the issue of family limitation, and finally separated. The Rev. Besant also was responsible for his wife's breaking away from Christianity.

Annie Besant continued her education after the collapse of her marriage. In 1879, following a period of tutoring by Dr. Edward Aveling,[30] a lecturer in comparative anatomy at London Hospital and sometime common-law husband of Karl Marx's daughter, Eleanor, Besant won admission to the South Kensington branch of London University. She read mathematics, physics, chemistry, and biology. She won honors in botany, where one of her examiners was Charles Darwin's defender, Thomas Huxley. Yet because of her atheism and public stance on such controversial issues as the legal rights of women and birth control, her attempts to obtain her B.Sc. degree were ultimately subverted by the male chauvinism of the day. Forty years later, the Benares Hindu University in India conferred on her the degree of Doctor of Letters *honoris causa* "for her tireless efforts

29. Ibid., p. 24.
30. Aveling was one of the "despicable types" of the Victorian age and thoroughly detested by the Marxists of his day, although he assisted in the translation of *Das Kapital* into English. Eleanor Marx, while living with him, learnt one day that he had secretly married someone else, whereupon Eleanor fatally shot herself.

in support of education and Home Rule for India." She had founded the Central Hindu College at Benares (now Varanasi) in 1898, the precursor of the present Benares Hindu University.

During her lifetime Besant spearheaded a number of campaigns and held responsible positions in various organizations. She was Secretary of the Malthusian League, the Neo-Malthusian organization in London that promoted the dissemination of birth control information. In 1878 she helped organize the International Labour Union. Ten years later, along with social democrat Herbert Burrows, she formed the Matchmakers' Union, after both had led a successful and orderly strike of girls working in match factories when the male-dominated British Trades Union refused to support their grievances. Her eloquent arguments as a lay woman lawyer in the custody hearings of her two children led to a revision of the government's policy of giving a father absolute rights over children. Through her journal, *Our Corner*, she helped launch the career of George Bernard Shaw. In 1885 Besant became one of the founders of the Fabian Society and worked hard as a speaker and writer on its behalf, her colleagues of the period being Sidney and Beatrice Webb, George Bernard Shaw, and Graham Wallace. She won election to the London School Board, where her achievements included a program of free meals for poor students and the institution of medical examinations and treatment in elementary schools.[31]

31. In 1889 Mrs. Besant appeared in the Court of Queen's Bench in a case that was given wide publicity. She sued the Rev. Edwyn Hoskyns, rector of Stepney, for damages in respect of an alleged libelous hand bill (published by him in 1888, when she was a candidate for election to the London School Board), contesting the division of the Board's area that included the parish of Stepney. In the hand bill, Hoskyns attacked Besant for her atheistic opinions and her advocacy of contraception, and made certain grave statements about her teaching, which he thought might justly be inferred from her writings. He caused the hand bill to be distributed at the doors of all the churches and chapels in his parish on the evening of Sunday, November 25, 1888, the day before the election.

Besant conducted her own case, and the Solicitor-General appeared for Hoskyns. When the Solicitor-General was reading extracts from a birth control publication, the jury suggested to the judge that the ladies present

She also worked tirelessly for the abolition of all child-labor abuses.

Long before she ever set foot in Ireland, she was one of the more ardent and vocal supporters of Irish home rule. When she embraced Theosophy at the persuasion of Madame Helena Petrovna Blavatsky (1831–1891), its founder, she went to India in 1893 and settled at Adyar, Madras, the world headquarters of the Theosophical Society, where she attempted a revival of Hindu culture and religion. When in 1907 she became president of the Theosophical Society, she not only organized and propagated its various activities but she also formed, in 1911, the Order of the Star of the East around her protégé, Jiddu Krishnamurti, a Telugu boy from Madras whom she proclaimed to be the new Messiah. She wrote little poems and essays and published them in his name. In 1915 Jiddu Krishnamurti's father, who was in difficult financial circumstances, entrusted the education of his two young sons to Besant. In 1926–1927 she traveled widely in England and the United States with Krishnamurti and eloquently urged his claims to be the new Messiah. On her return to India, she became involved in a law suit with the father of the boy over his custody and this incident largely reduced her prestige and popularity. In 1929 the young Krishnamurti, aware that Besant's claims for him were not valid, gathered sufficient courage to dissolve the Order of the Star of the East and repudiated the very idea of his messianic role.

Meanwhile, Besant diverted her energies to the cause of India's freedom. In 1916 she founded the Home Rule League, became its first president, and authored the Commonwealth of

---

should leave the court. The judge agreed, but added that he thought all the respectable ladies had already done so. The case was left undecided because the jury disagreed. The trial lasted four days, November 13–16, 1889. The hand bill, it seems, did not seriously damage Mrs. Besant's candidacy for the London School Board; she headed the poll with a majority of fifteen thousand. See G. F. McCleary, *Peopling in the British Commonwealth* (London: Faber and Faber, 1955), p. 49.

India Bill.[32] In 1917 she became president of the Indian National Congress (the present-day Congress party) at its Calcutta session. She was its fifth and last British president. Though she disassociated herself from the extremist section of the Indian National Congress, she was considered politically dangerous by the British government in India and was interned for some months of 1917. While the Montagu–Chelmsford reforms designed to further India's self-rule were under consideration, Besant at first supported the government, but after a brief spell of constitutionalism she began to support the extreme nationalist position. Soon she broke with Mohandas K. Gandhi, the rising star on the Indian political firmament, over his policies of *ahimsa* (nonviolence) and *satyagraha* (soul force). As history attests, Besant made a serious mistake, for it was Gandhi's unique methods that captured the imagination of the Indian people, broke down British imperialism, and eventually enabled India to regain her lost political freedom in 1947.

In the years after the end of World War I, both her political influence and that of the Theosophical Society declined to the point of almost ceasing to matter in Indian public life. She died at her Theosophical headquarters at Adyar, Madras, in 1933.

Before we examine Besant's role as an advocate of birth control, we may sum up her other contributions by saying that, although she was neither an original thinker nor particularly learned, she was a publicist and propagandist *par excellence*. Whatever cause she embraced and espoused, she gave it her wholehearted support and brought to bear on its furtherance all her considerable organizational skills and oratorical abilities. For

32. Besant was also one of the early champions of women's liberation in India. She was among those who inspired the founding of the Women's Indian Association in Madras and was its first president. She brought together able, educated Indian women from different parts of the country and voiced their pleas for a variety of reforms in an effort to influence Indian public opinion and the British government of the day in India. In this cause she was ably assisted by her less-known Irish colleague, Mrs. Margaret Cousins, wife of a minor Irish poet, Dr. James H. Cousins, who came to and settled in Madras at Besant's behest. Incidentally, Dr. Cousins embraced Hinduism, changed his name to Jayaram, and became a Theosophist.

example, when she came under the influence of Madame Blavatsky's views on reincarnation—views Besant expounded and embellished with her characteristic vigor when she succeeded Madame Blavatsky as president of the Theosophical Society (at Adyar, Madras, in 1907)—her genius as a propagandist and organizer brought to this occult society an influence far out of proportion to the numerical strength of its membership.

Apart from the esoteric ideas that formed a significant part of the Theosophical doctrine itself, Besant believed that Masters and Mahatmas in Tibet and the Gobi desert communicated with her. Perhaps that these regions were not adequately mapped geographically during her time tempted her to use them as the home of her mythical masters.[33] But while she gave thirty-four of her eighty-six years of life to Theosophy, we remember her here for what she did for Neo-Malthusianism and the battle she won with Bradlaugh.

2

After leaving her husband, Annie Besant endured many hardships and faced many difficulties, but none deterred her restless spirit. In 1874 she joined the National Secular Society and in that same year met Charles Bradlaugh. Soon she was given a job on Bradlaugh's *National Reformer* and joined forces with the radical politician and freethinker. Within a short period she rose to certain fame (or notoriety, from the mid-Victorian point of view) through her lectures on such subjects as "The Political Status of Women," "The True Basis of Morality," and "Civil

33. For an unintentionally amusing and entertaining version of the Theosophical-cum-clairvoyant view of anthropology, see Annie Besant and C. W. Leadbeater, *Man: Whence, How and Whither* (Madras: Theosophical Publishing House, 1913), p. 524.

While Besant was vigorously and vociferously advocating a revival of classical Hinduism, even to the extent of rationalizing its superstitions, her ignorance of the subject was considerable. Sometimes she made things up as she went along, e.g., "Dr. Besant tells us that the Spanish inquisitors were always reborn deformed. Where exactly she learned that one cannot tell"— S. Radhakrishnan, *An Idealist View of Life* (London: Allen and Unwin, 1957), p. 300.

and Religious Liberty," as well as her writings on these subjects.

Audiences in London and the provinces were soon being exhorted and harangued (and entertained) by this formidable intellectual and oratorical combination of Bradlaugh and Besant, with their progressive rationalist ideas that were so far ahead of the thinking of the times. It was, however, not easy sailing, for at times they had to suffer the hostility and even the occasional violence of unlettered crowds egged on by the obscurantist clergy.

Their eagerness to fight for just issues found a golden opportunity in Watts' prosecution for publishing Knowlton's book. With a sense of dedication and purpose they started the Free Thought Publishing Company behind Fleet Street and published Knowlton's banned book, *The Fruits of Philosophy*, in 1877.

In reissuing the book, Bradlaugh and Besant wrote a preface,[34] which clearly speaks for itself. Years later, while writing about her mentor and senior colleague, Charles Bradlaugh, Besant pointed out very briefly what really impelled them to publish the pamphlet, the same problem that brought and continues to bring most people to the subject of population control and family planning—poverty. She wrote: "We [Bradlaugh and Besant] recognized the horrible misconceptions that would probably arise; he [Bradlaugh] believed that he was forfeiting all hope of sitting [in Parliament] for Northampton; but the cry of the poor was in our ears, and we could not permit the discussion of the population question, in its own practical aspect, to be crushed. We did not like the pamphlet [*Fruits of Philosophy*] but to stop it was to stop all."[35]

## THE TRIAL

When the book was printed and bound, Charles Bradlaugh and Annie Besant deliberately invited arrest as a test case for publishing *Fruits of Philosophy*. In fact, Bradlaugh sent a copy

34. See pages 89–92 below.
35. Annie Besant, *Charles Bradlaugh: A Character Sketch* (Madras: Theosophical Publishing House, 1941), p. 52.

to the London police and informed them of the time and place when he and Besant would sell copies. Within a few days a plain-clothes detective bought a copy of the book for sixpence from Bradlaugh and the two social reformers were arrested on April 6, 1877, and tried before the Lord Chief Justice, Sir Alexander Cockburn, in June 1877.

But it is not clear who initiated the prosecution. Many suspected that an organization called the Society for the Suppression of Vice (which Besant sarcastically dubbed the "Society for the Promotion of Vice") was behind the incident. A few thought the Christian Evidence Society goaded the Home Secretary to arrest the two Neo-Malthusians. It was not the British government, nor the city authorities, nor any public agency or organization. Even the Lord Chief Justice wondered openly in the court who the prosecuting authorities were. In this connection Besant made the following observations during the trial:

It is one of the principles of English justice, that those accused shall be placed face to face with their accusers, and shall understand who brings them to answer before the bar of justice. Our difficulty in knowing the aim of the prosecution is, that we don't know at the present moment who is prosecuting us. When first we were arrested and taken to the Guildhall we were kept waiting for more than two hours shut up in the cold and uncomfortable cells under the Guildhall court of justice. We were then told that we were kept there to await the presence of the City Solicitor, who had the conduct of the prosecution. Hearing that, we thought we were to fight a prosecution conducted by the city authorities. We wrote to the City Solicitor, and our belief was strengthened by his answer, because the City Solicitor, writing on the paper of the Corporation, using the stamp of the Corporation, and signing under his name "City Solicitor," has only the right to use the funds of the city to conduct prosecutions for the city authorities; we naturally then believed that we were being prosecuted by the city authorities. Imagine our astonishment on Mr. Bradlaugh asking whether that was so, we were told that "the Corporation of the City of London has nothing and never had anything to do with the prosecution against you and Mrs. Besant"! ... We wrote to the solicitor and he wrote us telling us the Corporation had nothing to do with it, and referred us to the head of the Police of the city, who in his turn, in answer, said he had nothing to do with it, and that we must refer to the information. We found upon the information the name of William Simonds, there being no address given. We wrote for the address, which was furnished to us, and we then wrote to detective Wm. Simonds asking if he were the man responsible. We received in return merely an answer expressing his pleasure at receiving our letter.[36]

The trial lasted five days and went through several hearings and adjournments. The hearings took place at Guildhall. The press reported that large crowds assembled daily to witness the proceedings. Some contemporary witnesses estimated that more than 20,000 persons assembled outside the court. The sympathy of the public was obviously with the defendants.

While the prosecution was led by Sir Hardinge Gifford, the Solicitor General, Bradlaugh himself argued his defense in his usual masterly and studied manner, quoting from such authorities as Malthus, Fawcett, Mill, and Acton on population, economic, social and legal issues. He examined at some length the meaning and implications of the term "obscenity" in the context of Lord Campbell's Act, the Obscene Publications Act of 1857.

Besant then spoke for two days defending their action in publishing *Fruits of Philosophy*, much on the lines of their joint preface to the new edition of the book, and eloquently pleaded for limiting population growth in the context of England's socioeconomic situation. She concluded by referring to a "poor woman who had only 6 d. to spare and should be allowed to purchase with that 6 d. the knowledge which richer women can obtain for 2 sh. 6 p., 5 sh. or 6 sh. at any of the railway bookstalls of Messrs. Smith and Sons."[37]

Among the more prominent witnesses for the defendants were Miss Alice Vickery (who later became Mrs. Charles Robert Drysdale and President of the Malthusian League), Dr. C. B.

36. *In the High Court of Justice: Queen's Bench Division, June 18, 1877: The Queen v. Charles Bradlaugh and Annie Besant* (London: Freethought Publishing Co. [1877]), pp. 52–53.
37. Ibid., p. 36.

Drysdale, consulting physician to the Metropolitan Hospital, and Henry George Bohn, London publisher.

According to contemporary accounts, Bradlaugh and Besant received considerable support during the trial from various quarters, both within and outside England. Notable among their supporters were Emile Acollas, a French jurist; Touzzeau Parris, a prominent Bristol Unitarian minister; and General Guiseppe Garibaldi, the Italian political leader.[38]

Everyone who heard the defendants was impressed by their speeches, which revealed their knowledge of population problems and the pressing need for small families, as well as their knowledge of the intricacies of the law on obscenity.

The prosecution's case was not particularly impressive. Sir Hardinge Gifford observed, "I say that this is a dirty, filthy book, and the test of it is that no human being would allow that book on his table, no decently educated English husband would allow even his wife to have it. . . . The object of it is to enable a person to have sexual intercourse, and not to have that which in the order of providence is the natural result of that sexual intercourse. That is the only purpose of the book and all the instruction in the other parts of the book leads up to that proposition."[39]

The Solicitor General, Sir Hardinge Gifford, tried to convince the judge and jury that Dr. Knowlton had deceptively used Malthusian arguments as a pretext for suggesting promiscuous intercourse without the risk of pregnancy. However, he abandoned this approach after an indignant rebuke from the Lord Chief Justice, Sir Alexander Cockburn. Thereafter, the prosecuting counsel contented himself with declaring that it was ille-

38. Besant pointed out years later that "letters of approval and encouragement came from the most diverse quarters" including "letters literally by the hundred from poor men and women thanking and blessing us for the stand taken. Noticeable were the number of letters from clergymen's wives and wives of ministers of all denominations" (Annie Besant, *An Autobiography* [London: Unwin, 1893], p. 209).

39. *In the High Court of Justice*, p. 251.

gal to issue a work containing "a chapter on restriction, not written in any learned language, but in plain English, in a facile form, and sold . . . at sixpence."

Chief Justice Cockburn remarked, "A more ill-advised and more injudicious proceeding in the way of a prosecution was probably never brought into a court of justice. . . . I should very much like to know who are the authorities who are prosecuting, because that has not yet transpired. The Solicitor General tells us it may have been the Magistracy. I do not believe it."[40]

Sir Alexander summed up in favour of the defendants. After listening to the proceedings for five days, the jury returned a somewhat ambiguous verdict: "We are unanimously of the opinion that the book in question is calculated to deprave public morals, but at the same time we entirely exonerate the defendants from any corrupt motives in publishing it."[41]

The Chief Justice was therefore obliged to treat this opinion as a verdict of guilty, but he reserved judgment and allowed the defendants to go on their own recognizances. Later, when delivering the judgment, he declared that the defendants' whole attitude with regard to the book had been far from blameworthy, but he demanded their surrender of the book because it had been condemned by the jury. When Bradlaugh and Besant refused to do so and announced their intention to continue to sell the condemned book, the judge sentenced both to six months imprisonment, a fine of two hundred pounds, and recognizances of five hundred pounds for two years. However, on their giving notice of appeal, the execution of sentence was stayed. The judge allowed them to go on their own recognizances on condition that they did not try either to publish or sell the book until the appeal was heard and the verdict given. Besant's ironical comment on the verdict was that it amounted to saying, "Not guilty, but don't do it again."

In February 1878 the case came up on appeal. Bradlaugh and Besant moved for a writ of error and on this purely technical

40. Ibid., p. 255.
41. Ibid., p. 255.

ground (that the words relied upon by the prosecution were not expressly set out) the Court of Appeal reversed the judgment of the Queen's Bench and the sentence was quashed.[42]

But it should be pointed out that the judgment was far from a "victory or vindication of a principle,"[43] for it was based mainly on the technical inadequacies displayed in the prosecution's charge, regarding the words alleged to be obscene, which actually had not been set out. One of the appeal judges, L. J. Branwell, made this matter clear when he pointed out, "I wish it to be understood that we express no opinion whether this is a filthy and obscene, or an innocent book. We have not the materials before us for coming to a decision upon this point. We are deciding a dry point of law, which has nothing to do with the actual merits of the case."[44]

Thus Bradlaugh and Besant finally won the case. Earlier Bradlaugh had legally recovered from the police the seized copies of *Fruits of Philosophy*, which were sold after their winning the case, with the words "Recovered from Police" stamped across the cover of the book in red. They continued the sale of the book "till all prosecution and threat of prosecution were definitely surrendered" sometime in 1879.[45]

### THE TRIAL AND THE ENGLISH PRESS

As observed earlier, birth control propaganda in England did not begin with Bradlaugh and Besant, but was carried on during

42. The technicality on which the sentence was quashed rested on the fact that the statement on which the *Fruits of Philosophy* was adjudged obscene had not been specifically set forth during the trial, obviously an oversight. According to the Law Reports of the trial, "In an indictment for publishing an obscene book, it is not sufficient to describe the book by its title only, for the words thereof alleged must be set out; and if they are omitted the defect will not be cured by a verdict of guilty, and the indictment will be had either upon arrest of judgement or upon error." *The Law Reports: Queen's Bench Division, 1876–77* (Victoria, London) (1877) p. 607.
43. D. V. Glass, *Population Policies and Movements in Europe* (Oxford: Clarendon Press, 1940), p. 33.
44. 1878 L.R. 3 Q.B. 607 and 625, as quoted by D. V. Glass, p. 33.
45. Annie Besant, *An Autobiography*, p. 220.

the time of Francis Place, if not earlier. While some people knew of birth control and even practiced it, the propaganda in its favor, when permitted, was received with hostility by the church and state. But during and as a result of the trial, the atmosphere in favor of birth control changed radically. The public's reaction to the extensive daily coverage of the trial, with its flood of information, was not hostile but receptive at first and eventually accepting.

The English press—national and provincial—covered the trial in view of the mounting public interest. Most papers reported the proceedings in full and impartially reviewed the subject as news. At no time in British social history had the arguments in favor of a small family been presented so fully and freely. A few newspapers offered some editorial comment, both for and against the need for birth control. Yet this was a remarkable turning point, for until this moment no regular newspaper would touch the subject, much less endorse it, except a few radical organs of special groups like the freethinkers, Neo-Malthusians and secularists.

It is not necessary for our purpose to analyze the contemporary press coverage and comment in any detail.[46] A small and random sample will suffice to show which way the winds were beginning to blow.

A few papers gave verbatim reports of the speeches of the defendants, explaining their reasons in favor of family limitation. A few even presented extracts from Knowlton's book, while everyone knew that, paradoxically, the reason for the prosecution was for publishing "a certain indecent, lewd, filthy, bawdy, and obscene book called *Fruits of Philosophy*." *The Daily News* and *The Western Morning News* apparently belonged to this cate-

46. J. A. and Olive Banks have examined some fifteen national and thirty provincial newspapers of the day and have analyzed their coverage of the Bradlaugh–Besant trial. They found three national and ten provincial newspapers reported the trial without comment. Ten national and fourteen provincial newspapers reported the proceedings with unfavorable comment. And two national and six provincial newspapers reported with relatively favorable comment. See "The Bradlaugh–Besant Trial and the English Newspapers," *Population Studies*, 8, no. 1 (July 1954).

gory. The simple truth was that the trial was something of a surprise, and the readers' curiosity was apparently limitless.

A second group of newspapers gave adequate news of the trial but also gave their adverse editorial views. *The Times* led this group with bitter hostility. In fact, Besant pointed out later that the presence on the jury of Arthur Walter, son of the principal owner of *The Times*, was largely responsible for the verdict of guilty. *The Standard* and *Reynold's Newspaper* belonged to *The Times'* camp. *The Evening Standard* became imperialistic to the extent of pointing out that the Colonial Empire needed a large population: "It is not true that the world, or one hundredth part of it, is overpopulated."

A third group of newspapers had some latent sympathy for the cause, both in their editorial comments and in the special articles they ran. *The Daily Telegraph* felt convinced that population pressure was the major cause of poverty and granted the need for limiting family size but was not certain that this could be done by Knowlton's "vile work." In a similar vein the *Manchester Examiner and Times* conceded the need for birth control but felt compelled to advocate "moral restraint" or some kind of "prudence" and was against Knowlton's method of sponge and douche. *The Bradford Observer* admitted the nature of the problem and was sincere enough to recommend birth control to faraway India. It wrote:

No one can deny that the population question is one of extreme difficulty, or urgent importance in India, where we are staying the "natural checks" of famine, plague and war, and introducing nothing in their place; of urgent importance, too, at home where the population tends to increase faster than the means of subsistence. Here, then, is a vast and very difficult problem. The book which has been the subject of this trial, made an attempt—and an honest if mistaken attempt—to solve the problem. Say that the answer was ever so false; that the remedy proposed was worse than the disease; what then?[47]

47. *Bradford Observer*, June 23, 1877, as quoted in J. A. and Olive Banks, p. 30.

And last, the *Leicester Weekly Post*, which perhaps best reflected the changing tide of public opinion on the importance of the population and sex question, wrote that there was nothing wrong in discussing them:

We not only regret the prosecution, but we regret the verdict. The question of over-population and the checks to it is one that ought to be open to discussion. We do not say that it should be discussed in a public journal; the man who buys a newspaper buys it in order to get news, and has a right to expect that delicate topics like the one in question should not be brought before his children unawares. But that the matter is one which may fairly be argued, we do not see how there can be any doubt; and if so, and if the discussion is confined to books which are known to deal with it, so that a man buying any of them knows what kind of thing he is going to buy, we cannot see how public morals are injured. Of course it may be that a book written ostensibly with one object may be really written with another, and that an author professing to deal with a subject belonging to the range of physiology and political economy is really seeking to corrupt youth and to incite to vice. But this does not seem to have been chargeable against Knowlton and his book. The Lord Chief Justice expressly exonerated him from a charge of this kind, declaring it to be wholly unjust. Undoubtedly there are some minds which will find in the most strictly scientific treatise an incitement to lust; but they will do the same with many of the stories contained in the Old Testament, and unless we are prepared to prosecute the Bible Society for selling a book containing the stories of Joseph and Potiphar's wife, and of Amnon and Tamar, and half a dozen other narratives of the kind, we do not see the justice of the verdict which has been given against Mr. Bradlaugh and Mrs. Besant. This verdict seems to us, moreover, a very grave infringement upon the liberty of the Press, and that is, perhaps, the most serious point of the matter. If books may not be sold, of course they will not be written, and to condemn a man for selling a book dealing with a professedly open and arguable subject is to say that the subject ought not to be discussed in print. That was the position taken up some centuries ago by theologians; they in their day would have as vigorously prosecuted the man who wrote a treatise discussing the Trinity as the prosecutor in the present instance has prosecuted Mr. Bradlaugh and Mrs. Besant for selling *The Fruits of Philosophy*. Englishmen long ago made up their minds that all theological topics were open to question, and those who come after us will, we doubt not, in spite of the verdict in the present trial, contend that it is both lawful and expedient that sexual matters shall be open to discussion.[48]

With the enormous newspaper publicity that the trial received, the sale of *Fruits of Philosophy* in Great Britain jumped from about a thousand copies a year before the trial to more than 200,000 in the three-and-one-half years following it. The trial also resulted in such widespread public discussion and awareness of the issue of population growth and birth control outside England that in the following year, 1879, Dr. Aletta Jacobs, a Dutch woman physician, opened the world's first birth control clinic in Holland.

THE IMPACT OF THE TRIAL ON THE BRITISH BIRTH RATE

There is no doubt that the trial constituted a landmark in spreading the Neo-Malthusian view and more particularly contraceptive information to the poor and needy British working-class women. The daily publicity, even in the staid *Times* of London, not to speak of lesser and more sensational tabloids, that the trial received, the consequent general discussion of the pros and cons of birth control, including the actual knowledge of methods of controlling conception for which women were anxiously waiting, evidenced by the enormous sale of the book—all these affected the British birth rate. While this impact is generally accepted, there is some disagreement on the exact magnitude of the effect of the trial and whether some other not-so-obvious factors had also contributed to the dramatic and definitive decline in the British birth rate.[49]

To begin, the trial gave enormous publicity to *The Fruits of Philosophy*. While this little book had, as a piece of popular exposition, many defects compared to numerous later books, it became, faults and all, a best seller.

Second, the trial focused attention on contraceptive information as such. The information had already been available to the

48. *Leicester Weekly Post* June 23, 1877, as quoted in J. A. and Olive Banks, p. 30.
49. J. A. and Olive Banks, pp. 22–34.

educated, who believed that family limitation was not only permissible but socially desirable. And now the poor found that the information could be obtained legally, without hazard. The discussion of birth control acquired a new respectability, for the trial made it clear that "many important and respected personages did not regard family limitation necessarily as a set of 'indecent, obscene and immoral practices.' "[50] And above all, the spectacle of an educated and prominent woman, running the risk of ostracism and imprisonment, stoutly defending the right to discuss birth control, lent weight to the cause, and the taboo on birth control was broken. In a word, the trial marked the beginning of the democratization of birth control knowledge; that is, birth control information was made available to all—not just to the wealthy few.

To appreciate the trial and its much debated aftermath—the fall in the British birth rate—one must view it against the general socioeconomic background of the period. In England the onset of the Great Depression in 1874, ending a quarter-century of relative prosperity, compelled Britons to give up the things least necessary to them to maintain the decent level of living that they had achieved. Nothing seemed more superfluous than the unwanted child; for the Factory Acts that forbade the employment of children below the age of eight, and forbade children from eight to thirteen years of age to work more than half time, had made the British child—formerly a source of additional income to the family—now a source of some expenditure.[51] The financial burden of the child to the family was further increased by the passage of the Education Acts (Elementary Education Act, 1870; Education Act [Lord Sandon's Act] 1876; and Mundella Act, 1880), by raising the age for leaving school, coupled with a drop in the infant and child mortality rates.[52]

50. *Population Policy in Great Britain* (London: Political and Economic Planning, 1948), p. 67.

51. E. M. Elderton, *Report on the English Birthrate, Part I, England North of the Humber* (London: University of London, 1914).

52. Peter R. Cox, *Demography* (Cambridge: The University Press, 1950), p. 281.

During this period the social reformers went about preaching that couples had no right to have children unless they could adequately support them. This action countered to some extent the evangelical doctrine that "it is God who sends children and He will in due course provide for them." The working-class people and those belonging to the poorly paid professional classes began to realize that a large family became a handicap to "their progress as well as to their comfort." This was also the period when all aspects of the long-accepted moral, religious, and social dogmas and respectabilities of mid-Victorian England were being questioned. Many leaders in British public life helped diffuse a rationalist temper among the thoughtful of all classes that questioned traditionally accepted beliefs. And last, in the 1870s and 1880s, the intellectuals in England came to possess an almost fanatical faith in science and the scientific method and fervently believed that science, and science alone, could sweep away all human ills and misery. This new cult of the scientific method found supporters even in crowded working-class districts.

As for the actual impact of the trial on the British birth rate, there appear to be three views. According to the first, the trial's direct and telling effect was a rapid fall in the nation's birth rate. In England and Wales the average annual crude birth rate during the years 1871–1875 was 35.5 per thousand (which is roughly India's current birth rate) and it declined to 31.3 per thousand between 1886–1890. And from then on it went down steadily until it reached 15.0 per thousand in 1931–1935.

(Besides Knowlton's *Fruits of Philosophy* and Besant's *Law of Population*, many marriage and contraceptive manuals saw the light of day during the next few years and enjoyed wide circulation among the literate married women workers in the textile districts of Lancashire and West Reading. In these areas the English birth rate first began to fall. Birth control had become acceptable, respectable, and had come to stay.)

The second view gives the least importance to the trial for the falling birth rate. It contends that a significant fall in the birth rate of a community or a nation is too complex a demographic phenomenon to be the product of the proceedings of an English law court. In the view of some, contraceptive practices were being increasingly used in England and other countries, even before the 1870s, without the stimulus of a Bradlaugh–Besant trial.

In this connection, the report of the Royal Commission on Population pointed out the role of several fundamental forces:

The explanation lies, we think, in the profound changes that were taking place in the outlook and ways of living of people during the nineteenth century. The main features of these are well known. They include the decay of small-scale family handicrafts and the rise of large-scale industry and factory organization; the loss of security and growth of competitive individualism; the relative decline in agriculture and rise in importance of industry and commerce, and the associated shift of population from rural to urban areas; the growing prestige of science which disturbed traditional religious beliefs; the development of popular education; higher standard of living; the growth of humanitarianism and the emancipation of women. All these and other changes are closely inter-related; they present a complex web rather than a chain of cause and effect; it would be exceedingly difficult to trace how they acted and reacted on each other or to assess their relative importance.[53]

While these factors did operate and react with each other, they do not explain the sharp, dramatic fall in the birth rate immediately after the trial in 1877. Had the trial no direct and serious impact, the decline in the birth rate should have been gradual. Therefore, the third view—that the trial primarily and various other factors secondarily were responsible for the fall in the birth rate—appears to be reasonable under the circumstances.

The economic, social, and other fundamental forces were there; they might have even accounted for the ultimate circumstance causing the people to desire to limit the size of the family. But these forces would have mattered little in the absence of an event like the Bradlaugh–Besant trial. Of course, they created the necessary physical atmosphere. But without a corresponding mental and emotional atmosphere, the English people could not

53. United Kingdom, Royal Commission on Population, 1949, *Report* (London: H. M. Stationery Office, 1949), Cdm. 7695, rpt. 1953, p. 38.

have achieved the result. The trial, as pointed out earlier, democ-ratized the knowledge of contraception. It acted as a catalyst and crystallized public opinion in favor of birth control. Because of it, the other basic forces were able to bring about the fall in the birth rate.

The contention that the dramatic fall in the birth rate would have occurred had there been no Bradlaugh–Besant trial seems equivocal. In all probability the decline would have been postponed but for the trial and its publicity. James Alfred Field rightly points out:

In England particularly, as several careful studies have shown, the drop appears suddenly about 1878. The coincidence of this change with the propaganda called forth by the Bradlaugh–Besant trial is too significant to be ignored. The deeper causes of birth restrictions, of course, were latent in general social conditions. The falling birth rate would have come, no doubt, in its own time, had the *Fruits of Philosophy* never been protested. But the ill-starred prosecution gave to slow-gathering forces instant and overwhelming effect.[54]

### THE MALTHUSIAN LEAGUE (1877–1927)

A second important result of the trial, which was incidentally another factor that influenced the decline in the birth rate, was the rejuvenation of the Malthusian League. In 1877 the Malthusian League was started in London as the first voluntary organization in the world to advocate publicly limitation of the size of the family as the effective answer to poverty. The League's avowed objectives were:

1. To agitate for the abolition of all penalties on the public discussion of the Population Question, and to obtain such a statutory definition as shall render it impossible, in the future, to bring such discussions within the scope of the common law as a misdemeanor.

2. To spread among the people, by all practicable means, a knowledge of the laws of population, of its consequences, and of its bearing upon human conduct and morals.[55]

---

54. James Alfred Field, *Essays on Population and Other Papers* (Chicago: University of Chicago Press, 1931), p. 224.
55. Listed in all the issues of *The Mathusian,* the League's monthly journal.

It was the redoubtable Charles Bradlaugh who hit upon the idea of founding, or rather reviving, this organization at the height of his and Besant's trial. Bradlaugh had thought of creating this association much earlier, when he was constantly writing Neo-Malthusian articles in his journal, *The National Reformer*. And he had in fact started the organization in 1861, sixteen years before the trial, but somehow at that time it had not taken off.

In fact, Bradlaugh had been a Neo-Malthusian ever since he entered public life. In one of his lectures, delivered as early as 1852, he pointed out:

> There can be no permanent civil and religious liberty, no permanent and enduring freedom for humankind, no permanent and enduring equality amongst men and women, no permanent and enduring fraternity, until the subject which Malthus wrote upon is thoroughly examined and until the working men make that of which Malthus was so able an exponent the science of their everyday life; until, in fact, they grapple with it, and understand that the poverty which they now have to contend against must always produce the present evils which oppress them.[56]

However, it was the trial that gave a fillip to the Neo-Malthusian movement by attracting public support and finance and persuaded Bradlaugh to revive the defunct Malthusian League, this time with Dr. Charles Robert Drysdale (1829–1907) as president and Besant as secretary (until 1891, when she became a Theosophist and severed all her connections with Neo-Malthusian activities). When the League was formally inaugurated in July 1877, some 220 members enrolled in the very first week. And when President Drysdale started the League's slim monthly journal, *The Malthusian*,[57] with its subtitle, *A Crusade Against Poverty*, in February 1879, the first issue sold out in a week. The

---

56. Hypatia Bradlaugh Bonner and John M. Robertson, *Charles Bradlaugh: A Record of His Life and Work*, 5th ed. (London: Fisher Unwin, 1902), II, p. 172.

57. *The Malthusian* came out regularly from 1879 to 1921, and again from 1949 to 1952.

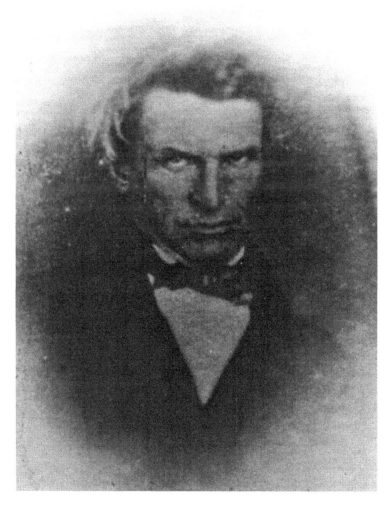

*Charles Knowlton, M.D., 1800–1850.*
*Courtesy of the Sophia Smith Collection, Smith College.*

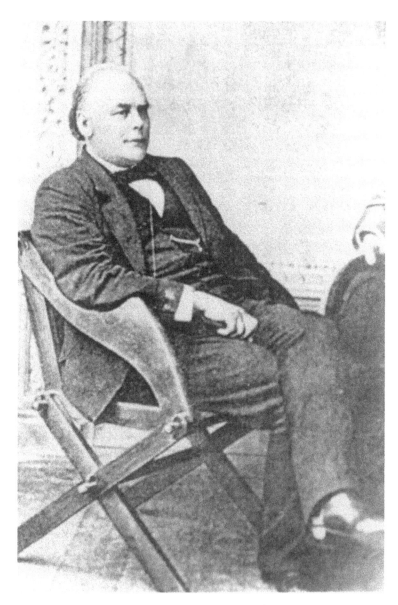

*Charles Bradlaugh, 1833–1891.*

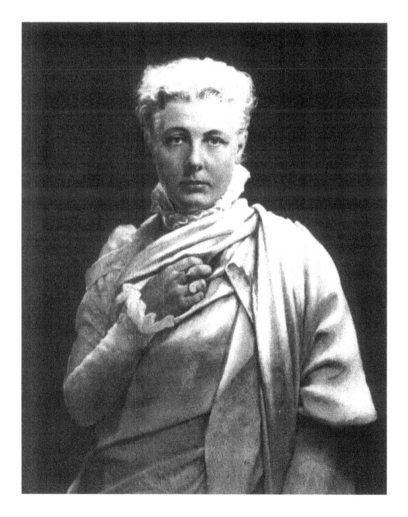

*Annie Wood Besant, 1847–1933.*

time for the dissemination of the Neo-Malthusian idea had arrived.

The new president of the League, Dr. Drysdale, was a Scottish physician in comfortable circumstances, brother of Dr. George Drysdale (1825–1904), another distinguished Neo-Malthusian physician and anonymous author of the widely used medical tome *The Elements of Social Science* (1854). In fact, the Drysdale family, including Dr. Alice Vickery (1844–1929), the able wife of Charles Drysdale, who succeeded her husband as president on his death in 1907, and their son, Charles Vickery Drysdale (1874–1961), rendered more dedicated and enduring service to the cause of Neo-Malthusianism than any other family group, for more than half a century donating their time, energy, intellectual zeal, and money to the cause without expecting any reward.

The League went about disseminating the Neo-Malthusian doctrine that a lowered birth rate and a small family were the cure for poverty and low wages. Members pleaded in popular lectures, penny pamphlets, and in their journal for limiting the family size on economic, health, medical, and social grounds.

In the beginning the movement's propaganda was confined to the socio-economic aspects of the population question, particularly the effect of a large family on the depressed and squalid living conditions of the working classes. There were many hundreds among the audiences and the readers who felt convinced of this relationship, but when they wanted to know what solution was being advocated there was panicky public reticence on the part of the lay and medical speakers and members of the League. There was no clinical instruction in birth control until 1881, when Dr. Drysdale opened a medical branch of the Malthusian League.

*The Malthusian* flourished for seventy years, from February 1879 until October 1949, although the parent organization, the Malthusian League itself, became virtually defunct in 1927. In 1942 the name of the League's journal was changed to *The New Generation*, though the contents and format hardly underwent any change.

The articles, news, and notes in the journal faithfully reflected the work and vicissitudes of the League. Much of the thinking of the physicians, social reformers, radicals, secularists, and socialists of the Victorian period on the issue of population and poverty can be found in its columns. Though it was primarily directed to the British working and middle classes, *The Malthusian* found its way beyond England to a few European countries and to certain parts of the British Empire, including India.

The League's membership was varied, though most were secularists and were, by and large, followers of Charles Bradlaugh and his *brand* of radical politics. The total membership never exceeded 1,224 in the peak year of 1879, and it never fell below 1,000. It must be added that the League and *The Malthusian* wielded more public influence than their numbers would warrant.

The League's rules, like those of most voluntary associations, provided for a president, vice-presidents, a corresponding secretary, a treasurer, a solicitor, auditors, and an executive council of twenty members elected by the membership. Over the years the League began to include among its vice-presidents some concerned foreigners who were sympathetic to the cause and who had been working on similar lines in their own countries, carrying on Neo-Malthusian propaganda after having been inspired by the British Malthusian League. In 1880 these included Dutch, French, Italian, and Indian nationals. The only one from the British Empire was Mr. Murugesa Mudaliar, from Madras, India, who became a vice-president in 1880.

The Malthusian League wished to initiate birth control programs in such countries as India, China, and Japan, particularly India, which was an important part of the Empire. But financial constraint was apparently the only barrier, for the limited funds available were used up for domestic programs. In 1903 the leaders of the League lamented, "We only wish that we had funds sufficient to send missionaries of our real gospel—glad tidings— to India, China and Japan."[58] The League's activities—both the

58. *The Malthusian,* 27, no. 2 (1903), 10.

journal and the pamphlets—were not received without some re-percussions in India. Obviously many copies were mailed to prominent citizens in major Indian cities.

The Malthusian League carried on regular correspondence with its vice-president in India, Mr. Mudaliar, who brought out *The Philosophic Inquirer* in Madras. In fact, *The Malthusian* announced in December 1880 that "efforts to combat the evils of overpopulation in India were already bearing fruit in that distant land."[59] In December 1882 another Indian Neo-Malthusian, Mr. Muthiah Naidu of Madras, wrote to Dr. H. A. Albutt, an English physician, friend of Dr. Drysdale and member of the Council of the League, informing him of the founding of a Hindu Malthusian League and requesting Albutt to be a patron. Dr. Albutt was one of the few medical men of the period who had the courage to offer open professional support to birth control. According to Naidu, "The principles and rules of the new organization" were to be "the same as those of the parent League in London to which we intend to affiliate."[60] Naidu gave the name of Mr. L. Narusu, secretary of the new League, and Mr. Mooneswamy Naiker, both of Madras, as the first members enrolled. It is not clear whether Naidu's Madras Malthusian League suffered an early demise or lost touch with the parent League in London, for *The Malthusian* unfortunately gives no further news of the Madras organization.[61]

We have in the pages of *The Malthusian* one more reference to the beginnings of the birth control movement in India. When an Indian birth control society was formed in Delhi in 1922, Professor Gopalji of Ranjar College, Delhi, reported the news to the English Neo-Malthusians and added, "Members of the Indian Birth Control Society congratulate the parent society in

---

59. Rosanna Ledbetter, *A History of the Malthusian League, 1877–1927* (Columbus: Ohio State University Press, 1976), p. 192. This is a well-researched and readable review of the Malthusian League and its activities.

60. Unfortunately, I have not been able to trace any details about Mr. Naidu—the name is rather common in Madras—or about his publication.

61. Letter to H. A. Albutt from Muthiah Naidu, dated December 13, 1882; cf. *The Malthusian*, no. 49 (February 1883), p. 389.

England for organising the International Neo-Malthusian and Birth Control Conference at London on July 11–14, 1922."[62]

The transition between the end of the Malthusian League in 1927 and the founding of the present-day Family Planning Association in England was brief. Several associations had sprung up in England in the inter-war period to promote birth control. These associations, led by divergent groups of physicians, social reformers, women leaders, radicals, and so on, agreed on the compelling need for birth control for British society but had vital ideological differences based on economic and social factors. However, in 1930 the National Birth Control Council was formed to coordinate the work of all organizations working to promote planned parenthood in England. Nine years later, on the eve of the Second World War, the council was renamed the Family Planning Association, which continues its useful activities to this day.

62. Rosanna Ledbetter, p. 192.

## The Writings of Annie Besant

### The Law of Population

During the course of the Bradlaugh–Besant trial, Besant dashed off her own pamphlet on population, *The Law of Population: Its Bearing Upon Human Conduct and Morals,* published in London in 1877.

Bradlaugh and Besant did not think highly of Knowlton's book because it was "largely out of date."[63] In 1881 she explained why she wrote her own pamphlet: "We published . . . Knowlton . . . to test the right of issuing cheap physiological knowledge, merely because that particular pamphlet had just been prosecuted. Having after hard struggle won the right, we dropped the particular book which had been forced on us . . . and issued the same information in a better form."[64]

Twelve years later, Mrs. Besant in her autobiography pointed out:

I wrote a pamphlet entitled *The Law of Population,* giving the arguments which had convinced me of its truth, the terrible distress and degradation entailed on families by overcrowding and the lack of necessaries of life, pleading for early marriages that prostitution might be destroyed, and limitation of the family that pauperism might be avoided; finally giving the information which rendered early marriage without these evils possible. This pamphlet was put in circulation as representing our view of the subject. . . . We continued the sale of Knowlton's tract [*Fruits of Philosophy*] for some time until we re-

63. This was presumably in relation to Knowlton's medical advice. The real reason apparently was that Knowlton focused on personal factors within the family for his contraceptive advice, while Besant tied her pamphlet to broad social and economic trends, and incidentally to a highly simplified Ricardian economic theory.

64. Annie Besant, *Henry Varley Exposed* (London, 1881), p. 15.

ceived an intimation that no further prosecution would be attempted, and on this we at once dropped its publication, substituting for it my *Law of Population.*[65]

Besant dedicated this pamphlet "to the poor in great cities and agricultural districts, dwellers in stifling court or crowded hovel, in the hope that it may point out a path from poverty, and may make easier the life of British mothers."

The pamphlet contained no new material. Besant examined various checks to population growth. In discussing the rhythm or safe-period method, she pointed out that "it was not certain" and hence was of doubtful value. And she gave precisely the wrong advice about the fertile and sterile periods in women, for she incorrectly assumed the safe period to be from the fifth to the fifteenth day of the menstrual cycle. (One wonders to what extent the birth rate might have been raised as a result of this erroneous information.)[66]

Besant believed *coitus interruptus* to be "absolutely certain as a preventive" and without injurious side effects, but she was not enthusiastic about it. The third method of contraception she examined was that in vogue at the time, namely, "syringeing with a solution of sulphate of zinc or of alum," but she noted that doing so had certain disadvantages involving "taste and feeling."

She wrote that the use of a vaginal sponge was to be preferred, and in later editions she also endorsed vaginal pessaries. There were additions based on the latest available knowledge as new editions appeared; by 1885, for instance, she added that the sponge should be soaked in a dilute quinine solution. In one of the last editions before she withdrew the book, her contraceptive recipe almost became modern, for she recommended a rubber cervical cap (the diaphragm which with vaginal jelly came into use at the beginning of the twentieth century) in place of the vaginal sponge, as both were "absolutely unobtrusive."

Besant, however, condemned abortion as a method of popula-

65. Annie Besant, *An Autobiography,* pp. 212–213.
66. See Jacob Oser, *Must Men Starve?* (London: Jonathan Cape, 1956), p. 32.

tion control. She also appealed to the members of the medical profession to devote some attention to this branch of reproductive physiology because further research was needed to produce a better and more acceptable contraceptive.

Within three years of its publication, this six-penny pamphlet had sold 40,000 copies. And by the time Besant gave up all her earlier causes and ideologies to embrace Theosophy in 1891 and withdrew her pamphlet, some 175,000 copies of *The Law of Population* had been sold. Thus the contraceptive information she provided enjoyed a vast circulation both in the United Kingdom and abroad, largely among the working-class population.

While the publication and circulation of Besant's pamphlet encountered no legal obstacles in Britain,[67] either from Lord Campbell's Act or the Post Office Act, it was subject to court action in Australia, but even there Besant eventually came out successful.

In 1888 an Australian bookseller in New South Wales was arrested, tried, and fined five guineas and costs for selling *The*

67. An unfortunate side effect of her pamphlet's publication as well as the notoriety caused by the trial was that it deprived her of the custody of her young daughter Mabel. Rev. Frank Besant, having failed in his first attempt in 1875 to obtain custody of their daughter, made a second, more carefully planned attempt in 1878, when the decision in the Bradlaugh–Besant case was pending in the court. Rev. Besant's plan was to include in Mrs. Besant's trial the charge of blasphemy against her. Despite the intimation sent to him that Mabel was ill with scarlet fever, Rev. Besant sent a notice through court for the custody of the child, his vindictiveness against his wife overpowering his concern for the welfare of his daughter. The charges leveled against Mrs. Besant were that she propagated atheism, associated herself with "an infidel lecturer and author" named Charles Bradlaugh, published the birth control pamphlet of Dr. Knowlton, and wrote a book, *The Law of Population.* The petition was heard by the then Master of Rolls, Sir George Jessel, who, according to Mrs. Besant, was "a man animated by the old spirit of Hebrew bigotry." Sir George denounced Mrs. Besant's Malthusian views "in a fashion at once so brutal and so untruthful as to fact . . ." and gave the custody of the child to Rev. Besant.

Sir George also refused to stay the order till the hearing of Mrs. Besant's appeal against his decision took place. Her appeal produced little effect beyond giving her the right to visit her children. Mrs. Besant, however, decided against visiting the children until they came of age. Eleven years later, in 1889, both Arthur Digby and Mabel chose to return to her.

*Law of Population.* His conviction, however, was set aside in December 1888 by the Senior Puisne Judge of the Supreme Court of New South Wales, Mr. Justice Windeyer.

Commenting on this trial in her *Autobiography,* Besant quoted at some length the Australian Supreme Court Justice's verdict: "The judgement was spoken at that time as a 'brilliant triumph for Mrs. Besant,' and so I suppose it was. The judge forcibly refused to be any party to the prohibition of such a pamphlet, regarding it as a high service to the community." His judgment is reproduced below.

So strong is the dread of the world's censure upon this topic that few have the courage openly to express their views upon it; and its nature is such that it is only amongst thinkers who discuss all subjects, or amongst intimate acquaintances, that community of thought upon the question is discovered. But let any one inquire amongst those who have sufficient education and ability to think for themselves, and who do not idly float, slaves to the current of conventional opinion, and he will discover that numbers of men and women of purest lives, of noblest aspirations, pious, cultivated, and refined, see no wrong in teaching the ignorant that it is wrong to bring into the world children to whom they cannot do justice, and who think it folly to stop short in telling them simply and plainly how to prevent it. A more robust view of morals teaches that it is puerile to ignore human passions and human physiology. A clearer perception of truth and the safety of trusting to it teaches that in law, as in religion, it is useless trying to limit the knowledge of mankind by any inquisitorial attempt to place upon a judicial Index Expurgatorius works written with an earnest purpose, and commending themselves to thinkers of well-balanced minds. I will be no party to any such attempt. I do not believe that it was ever meant that the Obscene Publication Act should apply to cases of this kind, but only to the publication of such matters as all good men could regard as lewd and filthy, to lewd and bawdy novels, pictures and exhibitions, evidently published and given for lucre's sake. It could never have been intended to stifle the expression of thought by the earnest-minded on a subject of transcendent national importance like the present, and I will not strain it for that purpose. As pointed out by Lord Cockburn in the case of the Queen v. Bradlaugh and Mrs. Besant, all prosecutions of this kind should be regarded as mischievous, even by those who disapprove the opinions sought to be stifled, in as much as they only tend more widely to diffuse the teaching objected to. To those, on the other hand, who desire its promulgation, it must be a matter of congratulation that this, like all attempted prosecutions of thinkers, will defeat its own object and truth, like a torch, 'the more it's shook it shines'.[68]

### RECANTATION AND *Theosophy and the Law of Population*

Besant continued to work in London for the Neo-Malthusian League, of which she was the secretary from the time it was founded in 1878, until she became a Theosophist. We may briefly recall that, once she was converted to Theosophy in 1891 by Madame Blavatsky, the Russian occultist, traveler, and writer, she withdrew from the Neo-Malthusian League and gave up her belief in its philosophy of birth control.

When two years later she settled in Madras, India, as the leading light and high priestess of the World Theosophical Society, she stopped printing her little book, *The Law of Population and Its Bearing Upon Human Conduct and Morals,* withdrew all remaining copies of the book, and even destroyed the plates lest it be reissued by some publisher without her permission. Theosophy, Besant had discovered, was incompatible with the Neo-Malthusian ideals of *The Law of Population.*

She not only recanted her belief in birth control and all that Neo-Malthusianism stood for, but she also gave up free thought and just about everything else she herself had once stood for. Her faith in and enthusiasm for her new beliefs overshadowed everything else. By advocating birth control where it was most needed, Besant could have contributed much to the welfare of the Indian masses through the auspices of the Theosophical Society; instead, she devoted her energy to a fruitless effort to kindle a religious renaissance, an effort that took her on questionable excursions into esoteric realms of occultism.

Theosophy was founded in 1875 in New York by Madame Helena Petrovna Blavatsky and an American Civil War veteran,

---

68. Annie Besant, *An Autobiography,* pp. 222–223. Also, *Ex parte* Collins, *Law Reports,* New South Wales, IX (1888).

Colonel H. S. Olcott. The movement's headquarters have been in Madras, South India, since 1878, though substantial branches existed in the United States (first in San Diego, California, and later in Wheaton, Illinois), England, and a few other countries. Its activities—religious, cultural, and political—were confined to and concentrated in India for the first quarter of the century until Theosophy, both as a cult and a movement, ceased to have any relevance to India or the world.

The movement's aim was

"the establishment of a real brotherhood amongst all peoples which was held dependent on an esoteric ancient wisdom, expressed in the Vedanta and transmitted through 'Masters' or 'Mahatmas' who appear from age to age. These 'great souls' have occult powers which give them unique control over their own bodies and other natural forces. Under their guidance, humanity bound to the ever-turning wheel of reincarnation by the Law of *Karma,* will someday gain happiness in a world which will drink as one from the wonderful fountain of wisdom from which all religions have drawn their hitherto partial truths." In practice the Theosophists have defended prophecy, second sight, Hindu idol worship and caste with little critical discrimination between ideas.[69]

To explain her conversion to Theosophy and her consequent recantation of her belief in birth control, Besant brought out in 1896 a twenty-page pamphlet, *Theosophy and the Law of Population.* Here she faltered. The pamphlet fizzled like a damp squib. Whatever was thought of Theosophy and its "esoteric Mahatmas from the ethereal regions" from the religious and spiritual points of view, fortunately no one but fellow Theosophists paid much attention to Besant's new, Theosophy-oriented view on the population question.

The pamphlet reveals that her new-found spiritualism had vitiated her understanding of the basic postulates of the population issue, particularly in the poor and exploited country where she was living, and in the world at large, of which she had con-

69. As quoted in John B. Noss, *Man's Religions* (New York: Macmillan, 1967), p. 300.

siderable knowledge compared to her provincial Theosophical compatriots at Madras.

One is certain that Besant had read Malthus before she and Bradlaugh entered the fray by publishing Knowlton's book. There is no doubt that she understood the pressing economic and social parameters of the population problem and was aware of the impending population explosion in India that would compound the country's traditional, all-pervading poverty. But her commitment to Blavatsky's new nostrum of Theosophy was so complete and compelling that her better judgment and right instincts somehow failed her. The relevance of Theosophy to the population question was obvious only to a handful of true believers.

It must, however, be said to Besant's credit that her intellectual integrity must be commended in explaining the embrace of a new belief that was contrary to all that she had previously stood and fought for, and whose founder, Madame Blavatsky, was freely talked of as a fraud. Besant was a woman who always had the courage of her convictions, no matter how peculiar those convictions sometimes appeared.

True to Besant's life, there was to be still another surprise, this time a final one. When she wrote her last pamphlet on the population question, *Theosophy and the Law of Population,* it was taken by all concerned, Theosophists and others, both in India and England, as her final statement on the subject. But a few years later, at the turn of the century, she once again changed her mind and returned to the Neo-Malthusian view set forth in her earlier writings.[70] We may, therefore, suppose that Annie Besant died believing in both birth control and reincarnation.

According to the orthodox Theosophical view, there can be no population explosion, for the world's population does not grow. On the contrary, the total numbers are fixed and stand at a constant, stationary figure. The reasoning is simple, if irrational. A

70. Annie Besant, *An Autobiography*, pp. 318, 335–342; also see Hypatia Bradlaugh Bonner and J. M. Robertson, *Charles Bradlaugh: A Record of His Life and Work*, II, 19.

birth is not necessarily an addition for it is compensated by death. Everyone is reborn after death and because of the transmigration of souls, the cycle goes on forever. Even if there are more births than deaths, they even up eventually, for some souls take time to be reborn. Therefore, there is no such thing as burgeoning population growth. There is thus no need for birth control. The argument is so esoteric and irrational that one need go no further by raising any logical questions.

Annie Besant died in 1933 at her Theosophical home in Adyar, Madras. She had been a member of the organization for some forty-two years and was its president from 1907 on. As president of the movement she was succeeded by lesser and lesser individuals who shared neither her intellectual, organizational, nor communication gifts—nor her vision, such as it was. With the passing of years, Theosophy at first declined and then virtually disappeared from the Indian and international scene, while the magnitude of the population problem, both in India and the rest of the world, began to increase steadily until it became one of the modern world's intractable problems.

The slight and wavering flame lighted by Knowlton in the United States in 1832 had become in the 1930s a steady blaze, when a significant segment of European, American, and even some Asian women, had taken to contraception. Incidentally, the world's population, which reached the first billion about the time of the appearance of Knowlton's book, had doubled by the time of Besant's death.

Within a quarter-century of her death, birth control, or family planning, to give it its modern name, had become in one way or another an integral part of the health, economic, and social policies of nearly one hundred governments—a great majority of the member states of the United Nations.

As for scientific contraception, tremendous advances have been registered. The world has come a long way since Knowlton recommended a vaginal douche with vinegar. We have had the diaphragm and spermicidal jelly of the 1930s and 1940s, the IUDs of the 1950s, and the vasectomy, tubectomy, and "the pill" of the present day. (To these have been added women's right to abortion, which has been made almost routine thanks to the vacuum aspirator.) Spectacular possibilities of simple, cheap, harmless, and effective methods of conception control such as immunization, a monthly pill for males, and other variants are on the horizon. And the day is not far off, perhaps before the end of this century, when *every* child, all over the world, can be a wanted child, one loved and adequately cared for.

And thus a century after the Bradlaugh–Besant trial, when the world population has crossed the four-billion mark, we recall the significant court battle for the spread of an idea whose time had come. Today, thanks to the Bradlaugh–Besant court battle and the advent of modern contraception, the world has become a little better place in which to live, where women can, by and large, have babies by design and not by accident. The biological emancipation of women has come to stay.

# APPENDIX: NOTES ON INDIVIDUALS AND TERMS

## HELENA PETROVNA HAHN BLAVATSKY (1831–1891)

The Russian occultist and founder of the Theosophical Society, Madame Helena Blavatsky, was born in Russia of a German nobleman settled in Russia. Married in her seventeenth year to a Russian military man much her senior and separated from him after a few months, she traveled extensively in Europe, the Middle East, India, Tibet, and Java during the 1850s. She returned to Russia but again, in the late 1860s, traveled widely, particularly in Asia.

In 1873 Madame Blavatsky went to New York City where, with the assistance of Colonel Henry Steel Olcott, a Civil War veteran; William Q. Judge; and others she founded the Theosophical Society in 1875.

In 1879 she and Colonel Olcott went to India, and in 1883 they established the permanent headquarters of the Theosophical Society at Adyar, Madras.

Blavatsky's works include *Isis Unveiled* (1877), *The Secret Doctrine* (1888), *The Voice of Silence* (1889), and *The Key to Theosophy* (1889). Her *Collected Writings* were published by the Theosophical Society at Adyar in seven volumes, completed by 1958.

Madame Blavatsky claimed spiritual powers, but a representative of the Society for Psychical Research in London found no evidence of her "miracles," many of which were demonstrated to be fradulent in 1884. Before her death she converted freethinker Annie Besant to Theosophy.

## JEREMY BENTHAM (1748–1832)

Bentham, an English jurist and political philosopher, graduated from Oxford in 1766 and though called to the bar in 1772, did not practice. He studied the population problem in connection with his enquiry into the Poor Law question (1797–1798). Bentham was a friend of the Rev. Joseph Townsend (1739–1816), a Methodist clergyman, utilitarian, traveler, and author of *A Dissertation on the Poor Laws* (1786). Townsend is said to have brought Bentham the information that the vaginal sponge was used by French women to control conception. Bentham not only gave this information to Place and Carlile, but persuaded them to publicize it among the working classes while he remained in the background.

Although he is little known for his role in encouraging the spread of birth control information, he is famous as the author of *Introduction to the Principles of Morals and Legislation,* wherein he expounds his philosophy that morality of action is determined by utility: "that is, the capacity for rendering pleasure or preventing pain, according to which the object of all conduct and legislation is the 'greatest happiness of the greatest number.' "

## RICHARD CARLILE (1790–1843)

An English journalist, freethinker, and birth control propagandist, Carlile began as a chemist's boy and tinsmith's apprentice. Ambitious to earn a living as a writer, he hawked the radical paper *Black Dwarf* (1817–1824) for awhile till he was attracted to W. T. Sherwin and his *Sherwin's Weekly Political Register.* On Sherwin's marriage, Carlile took over his publishing business and became the editor of the radical *Register.*

When William Hane, a bookseller, published a parody of the Book of Common Prayer and other religious subjects, Carlile published them, as well as a series of his own imitations of them, while Hane was still in prison awaiting trial for blasphemy. For this Carlile was jailed for eighteen weeks. Later he began to republish Thomas Paine's *The Rights of Man* (1791–1792) and *The Age of Reason* (1794–1807). This action led to his second imprisonment and was the beginning of a series of imprisonments, for blasphemy and other offenses, totaling nine years and four months. But during his days in jail, he continued to edit his papers and his Fleet Street shop was managed successfully by his wife; and when she was imprisoned, by her sister, and so on. While Carlile was in jail his religious views underwent a change from Zeteticism (free infidel inquiry) to extreme materialistic atheism.

In 1825 Carlile reprinted Place's birth control hand bills in his journal, and encouraged by their reception, the next year he reprinted his own articles on *What Is Love?* as an anonymous pamphlet with the title *Every Woman's Book or What Is Love?*

After reviewing the then-available methods, it recommended the condom as the best contraceptive method. The pamphlet went into three reprintings within a year and some five thousand copies were sold. In 1829 Eliza Sharples became his common-law wife and bore him a daughter, Hypatia, in 1830.

### ANTHONY COMSTOCK (1844–1905)

A mistaken and misguided American moralist and reformer, Civil War veteran, clerk and dry-goods salesman, Comstock became involved with the Y.M.C.A. in a crusade against pornographic literature. He became a special inspector for the New York City Post Office and helped organize the New York Society for the Suppression of Vice. Under its auspices he worked vigorously to prosecute "criminal offenders," a term that included, according to him, "poets, writers, artists, physicians, abortionists, quack doctors, advertisers of contraceptives, etc." In 1873 Comstock managed to push a bill through an absentminded, puritanical Congress tightening the 1872 Act that prohibited the mailing of obscene matter. This bill defined information on "the prevention of conception" as obscene. This came under Section 211 of the Federal Criminal Code, which provided a maximum penalty of five years of imprisonment and a fine of $5000, exorbitant for those days, for anyone who sent through the U.S. mails any " 'paper, writing, advertisement or representation that any article, instrument, substance, drug, medicine, or thing may, or can be, used or applied, for preventing conception,' or any 'description calculated to induce or incite a person to so use or apply any such article, instrument, substance, drug, medicine, or thing' " (Mary Ware Dennett, *Birth Control Laws* [New York, 1926]).

Comstock worked incessantly—through raids, decoys, and publicity, and the entrapment of anyone even remotely suspected of informing the public even about the human anatomy. He was responsible for the arrest of nearly four thousand persons, of whom some three thousand were convicted and several committed suicide. He was also responsible for the trial of the crusader for women's rights Victoria Chaflin Woodhull for the "crime of exposing a love affair between a cleric, Henry Ward Beecher, and a parishoner wife." He even instituted legal proceedings against George Bernard Shaw's play *Mrs. Warren's Profession* in 1905. But Shaw and others had already begun to ridicule "Comstockery" as a disparaging term for puritanical crusading. In 1915 he arrested William Sanger, Mrs. Margaret Sanger's husband, for "selling" a copy of Mrs. Sanger's *Family Limitation*. Comstock died unlamented during Mr. Sanger's trial.

### MARIE-JEAN-ANTOINE-NICOLAS CARITAT, MARQUIS DE CONDORCET (1743–1794)

Condorcet was a noted French philosopher, mathematician, and politician. He was a member of the French Legislative Assembly (1791) and later its president (1792). He was a member of the National Convention and of the Girondists (moderate republican party in the French Legislative Assembly, 1791–1793). An anti-Jacobin, he was arrested with other members of the Girondist group. Before his death in prison, he completed his utopian book, *Esquisse d'un tableau historique des progrès de l'esprit humain* (1795). As philosopher of the French Revolution he envisioned a utopia in which man would attain eventual perfection. This book, when published in England, influenced British thought on the ultimate perfectibility of man. (Malthus's essay was an attempt at a refutation of Condorcet's *Esquisse*.)

As a mathematician, Condorcet made some notable contributions to the theory of probability.

### BENJAMIN FRANKLIN (1706–1790)

American printer, author, inventor, scientist, diplomat, and public official, Benjamin Franklin was born in Boston but settled in Philadelphia, where he obtained employment as a printer. He later became the proprietor of a printing and publishing business. He published *The Pennsylvania Gazette* (1730–1748) and edited *Poor Richard's Almanac* (1732–1757). He was appointed Deputy Postmaster General for the Colonies (1750–1774). He was a member of the Continental Congress and signed the Declaration of Independence. He spent nine years in France during the revolution as an American agent and was appointed Plenipotentiary to France in 1778. He helped negotiate the peace treaty with England.

In his famous kite experiment, Franklin proved that lightning is an electrical phenomenon. He improved the heating stove, which came to be called the Franklin stove (though he did not patent it). He helped reorganize the postal system, and improved street cleaning and lighting. He established the first circulating library in America. In 1751 he started the Academy of Philadelphia, which later became the University of Pennsylvania. In 1790 he signed a memorial to Congress asking for the abolition of slavery.

Besides his *Autobiography,* considered a classic of early American literature, he brought out a pamphlet, written in 1751 and published four years later, titled *Observations Concerning the Increase of Mankind and the Peopling of Countries.* He predicted the doubling of the population of the American colonies about every twenty years and anticipated by nearly half a century some issues of the later arguments of Malthus. Malthus quotes from Franklin's pamphlet in the second edition of his *Essay* (1803). Franklin published in 1760 a tract on a related subject titled *The Interest of Great Britain Considered with Regard to Her Colonies and the Acquisition of Canada and Guadaloupe.*

## WILLIAM GODWIN (1756–1836)

English philosopher, political theorist, and novelist, Godwin began as a cleric (1777–1782) but turned dissenter and atheist and devoted himself to study, literature, and writing. He dabbled unsuccessfully for some years in a publishing business (1805–1822). He wrote *An Enquiry Concerning Political Justice*

(London, 1793) and in this work propounded the utopian doctrine that experience shapes people according to certain rational principles, the only artificial barriers to which are the institutions of marriage, the class system, and organized government. This major work brought him certain fame as the philosophical representative of the English radicalism of the day. It may be recalled that Malthus wrote his famous anonymous essay on the Principle of Population to refute Godwin's utopian thesis. In answer to Malthus, Godwin brought out *Of Population* in 1820.

In later years Godwin modified his views on marriage and opposed the elopement of his daughter Mary with poet Percy Bysshe Shelley (1792–1822), who had been greatly influenced by Godwin's liberal and reformed views. Godwin was the author of a few novels as well as various miscellaneous works.

### AUSTIN HOLYOAKE (1826–1874)

Holyoake was the younger brother of George J. Holyoake. Austin, printer, publisher, and freethought lecturer, wrote a pamphlet entitled *Large or Small Families* (1870), which advocated birth control by the "safe" period method. He had earlier published Knowlton's *Fruits of Philosophy* without any encounter with the law. He also pleaded for a republican form of government for England.

### GEORGE JACOB HOLYOAKE (1817–1906)

English social reformer and lecturer on freethought and Owenite socialism, George Holyoake was the founder of secularism in Great Britain, of which movement Charles Bradlaugh became the leading light a few years later. Born in Birmingham, he taught mathematics for some years at the Birmingham Mechanics Institution. He raised funds and a contingent to aid Garibaldi in Italy. From 1846 he edited for a number of years a weekly called *The Reasoner,* which was devoted to freethought, socialism, and republicanism. He promoted the bill legalizing secular affirmation. Holyoake was the last person imprisoned in England for atheism (1842). He wrote on secularism, histories of the Cooperative Movement, and *Sixty Years of an Agitator's Life* (1892).

## JIDDU KRISHNAMURTI (1891– )

Indian Theosophist and philosopher, Krishnamurti was born in Madras, India. His father entrusted his and his brother's education to Annie Besant. He was educated in England by tutors and by Besant, who proclaimed him the Messiah in 1925. She founded The Order of the Star in the East to sustain her claim that Krishnamurti was the answer to all those who believed in the Second Coming. Later he dissolved The Order and retired. He lives in California and travels to India and other parts of the world, talking of his brand of the "religion" mankind needs. He is the author of a number of books.

## JAMES MILL (1773–1836)

James Mill, a Scottish philosopher, historian, economist, and East India Company official in England, was the son of a shoemaker and the father of John Stuart Mill. Mill was the founder of philosophic radicalism, and became editor of the *St. James Chronicle* in 1805 and a regular contributor to the *Edinburgh Review* (1803–1813). He met Jeremy Bentham in 1808 and became his close friend and an exponent of his utilitarian philosophy in England. Mill was appointed an official of the East India Company in 1819. He was among those largely responsible for the founding of the University of London in 1825.

While he wrote several books, Mill's magnum opus was *Analysis of the Mind* (1829) wherein he provides a psychological basis for Bentham's utilitarianism. He labored on his *History of India* for twelve years. His *Fragment on Mackintosh* (1835) contended that morality is based on utility.

## JOHN STUART MILL (1806–1873)

John Stuart was the precocious and brilliant son of James Mill, the Scottish philosopher, historian, and economist. The young Mill was given such a rigorous and systematic education that, when ten years old, he could read and comprehend what a normal twenty-five-year-old found difficult.

He became interested in the nation's population question as a youngster, when he saw the strangled body of a newborn baby in a London park, and later at seventeen, when he was recruited by Place to distribute his birth control hand bills to scullery maids and to the wives and daughters of tradesmen. A hostile crowd who noticed what John Stuart Mill and his young companions were distributing dragged them before a London magistrate, who sentenced them to a fortnight's imprisonment. But influential friends and family convinced the authorities that Mill's attempt to prevent infanticide (by controlling births) was not the promotion of obscenity. They were released after a few days and the matter was hushed up, but the incident was raked up half a century later by *The Times* in an obituary notice of Mill, whereupon Prime Minister Gladstone withdrew his promised support from a proposal for a public memorial to Mill. The subject of family planning was so sensitive that even a British Prime Minister did not have the moral courage to come out openly in support of such a distinguished Briton as Mill.

Like his father before him, Mill entered the service of the East India Company. He became a junior clerk in India House (1823), assistant examiner (1828) in charge of the Company's relations with India's princely states (1836–1856), and chief of office in 1856. He retired with a pension in 1858, when the East India Company was dissolved and the administration of India was taken over by the British government.

He was the author of *Principles of Political Economy* wherein he took a Neo-Malthusian view of the population question (third edition, 1852). His best-known work is *On Liberty* (1859), a treatise written against the background of British religious bigotry. He was one of the foremost defenders of the freethinkers in their struggle for civil rights.

He was a Member of Parliament for Westminster (1865–1868) and voted, with the advanced radical party of the day, for women's suffrage among other issues. On ceasing to be a Member of the House, he returned to his literary pursuits and brought out the *Subjection of Women* (1869) and his *Autobiography* (1873).

## NEO-MALTHUSIANISM

The term Malthusianism was used incorrectly in Great Britain and overseas for nearly half a century (from about 1850) to define a concept that is strictly Neo-Malthusian, which term came into vogue about the end of the nineteenth century. Neo-Malthusianism may be defined as the "theory" that accepts the Malthusian fears about the danger of overpopulation while rejecting Malthus's proposed solution of moral restraint—involving postponement of marriage until a couple was able to support children—as being unrealistic. Instead, Neo-Malthusianism advocates the practice of birth control within marriage, in the sense of various modern scientific contraceptive methods, a solution unacceptable to Malthusian theory.

## ONANISM OR COITUS INTERRUPTUS

The ban on the use of contraceptives among the orthodox Jews and Christians was based on a passage in Genesis 38:2–10. According to the narrative, Jacob's son Judah fathered three sons. The firstborn, Er, married Tamar but died young, leaving his wife childless. Thereupon Judah asked his second son, Onan, to "go into your brother's wife, and perform the duty of a brother-in-law to her, and raise up offspring for your brother." But when he did so, Onan "spilled the semen on the ground, lest he should give offspring to his brother." The act "was displeasing in the sight of the Lord, and He slew him."

According to the Jewish customary law, a brother was obliged to marry and beget children by his brother's widow. Early church leaders interpreted the passage as God's prohibition of contraception. Onan, having thwarted the natural end of sexual union, was considered to have sinned in God's eyes and was accordingly slain for his transgression—hence the Biblical disapproval of onanism, or coitus interruptus. However, the method has been one of the most popular and effective methods of birth control through the ages, particularly in Western culture.

## ROBERT OWEN (1771–1858)

Robert Owen was a wealthy Welsh manufacturer, pioneer of the Cooperative Movement, philanthropist, and Utopian socialist. He bought the New Lanark textile mills at Manchester with William Allen, Quaker philanthropist, and Jeremy Bentham as partners (1814). In his manufacturing establishment he stopped the employment of children and established sickness and old age insurance and recreational facilities for his workers. Exhausting much of his cotton-mill fortune, he founded several utopian "Owenite" communities in Great Britain and the United States, including one at New Harmony, Indiana (1825–1828). He was interested in birth control and was reported to have brought to England literature concerning the subject from France and other countries. While this was not substantiated, he was bitterly attacked for his free thought. He was the author of *A New View of Society* (1813), wherein he expounded his belief that a man's character and personality are largely determined by environment and human society, and can be improved by endeavors based on cooperative principles. He was the father of Robert Dale Owen.

## ROBERT DALE OWEN (1801–1877)

A pioneer in birth control in England and the United States, eldest son of Robert Owen, the affluent Welsh utopian socialist, Robert Dale Owen was educated privately in Scotland and Switzerland. His first job was that of superintendent of the school at his father's model "community" at New Lanark in Scotland, which assignment resulted in his first published work, *An Outline of the System of Education at New Lanark* (1824).

In 1821 Robert Dale accompanied his father to the United States, where the senior Owen was launching a new community based on rational education and cooperation at New Harmony, Indiana. There he edited *The New Harmony Gazette* (1825–1828). When the New Harmony experiment folded, he settled in New York and edited *The Free Enquirer* (1828–1835), and for a time during the 1830s *The New York Sentinel and Working Man's Advocate*.

As a result of certain curious circumstances wherein Richard Carlile's *Every Woman's Book* was published in his name, Owen had to make public his view that he was not opposed to Carlile's book; and two years later, in 1831, he brought out his own work, *Moral Physiology; or a Brief and Plain Treatise on the Population Question,* a seventy-two-page pamphlet recommending coitus interruptus and condoms. The essay is more a plea for family limitation for socio-economic reasons than a description of actual methods. The tract's importance was that it influenced the thinking of Dr. Charles Knowlton. The book was successful and went through nine editions in five years.

He served in the Indiana Legislature (1836–1838), was elected a member of the U.S. House of Representatives (1843–1847), and was U.S. minister to Italy (1855–1858). He was a lukewarm advocate of the emancipation of Negro slaves. His books include *The Policy of Emancipation* (1863), *The Right of Emancipation and the Future of the African Race in the United States* (1864), *The Wrong of Slavery* (1864), and *Threading My Way* (an autobiography) (1874).

### RHYTHM OR SAFE-PERIOD METHOD

The rhythm or safe-period method of birth control through periodic continence is based on the biological fact that conception is possible only on certain days of the woman's menstrual cycle when the mature ovum is released from the ovary into the fallopian tube. If coitus is avoided during the fertile period when the ovum is in place, conception can be (theoretically) avoided.

It is, however, not easy to determine the exact fertile and sterile days in a woman's cycle. Today, thanks to the early work of two physicians, Kyasaku Ogino of Japan and Hermann Knaus of Austria, the fertile, or rather, fecund period is placed at roughly "fourteen days *before* the onset of menstruation." That is, a few days immediately after menstruation may be considered the safe period. This calculation is based on body temperature and blood enzymes and can be ascertained relatively correctly for women with absolutely regular menstrual periods.

For ten years the government of India with the aid of the

World Health Organization of the UN advocated the rhythm method for a certain select population of married women and found it did not work, for women in sexual matters refused to be slaves of the calendar and the thermometer. There are apparently more failures than successes with this method.

The Catholic Church, which is the one major world religion still opposed to contraception, apparently approves of this method. But the Catholic doctrine on the subject is in flux, and a majority of the Catholics all over the world, according to the available evidence, apparently do not follow the papal dictum on sex.

### Nassau William Senior (1790–1864)

Senior was a well-known English economist of his day who held the first Chair of Political Economy at Oxford University. He conducted for the government some studies on contemporary economic conditions in England and helped frame the Poor Law of 1834. His *Two Lectures on Population* was published in 1828 (reprinted by Arno Press, New York, 1976).

### Shakers

A popular name for the members of the United Society of Believers in Christ's Second Appearance, the Shakers were also called the Millennial Church, based on the thousand years mentioned in Revelations during which holiness is to prevail and Christ is to reign on earth. The name "Shakers" was derived from the trembling caused by religious emotion that the Believers evidenced.

The early Shakers originated in England in 1747 during a Quaker (Society of Friends) revival led by James and Jane Wardley, and became known as the Shaking Quakers. The movement grew strong when a member, Ann Lee, professed to be the mother element in the Spirit of Christ and was imprisoned for her belief as well as for her zeal.

Directed by a vision, Ann Lee and a few followers emigrated to New York State in 1774 and established a colony near Albany in 1776. During the next half-century, Mother Ann, as she came to be known, gained numerous adherents and established eighteen Shaker settlements (or communities) in eight states between New York and Indiana. The Shaker villages were strict, celibate, communistic communities.

Singing, marching, and dancing marked phases of Shaker worship. During their dances the worshipers formed separate lines by sexes, and although the movements were ecstatic, there was no physical contact among the men and women. In church, men and women entered by separate doors and sat facing each other, betraying no emotion. Some members formed amorous attachments and eloped. Strict celibacy was responsible for the disappearance of the community, for they left behind no progeny and recruitment of new converts gradually ceased.

### EDWARD TRUELOVE (1809–1899)

A prominent English freethinker, Owenite socialist, and champion of male suffrage, Truelove was a publisher and bookseller. He was imprisoned for four months with a fine of fifty pounds when he was sixty-six years old for publishing Owen's *Moral Physiology*. When Dr. George Drysdale (whose pen name was G. R.), the Scottish physician, could not find a publisher for his controversial book on sex, *The Elements of Social Science,* Truelove offered to publish it in 1854. It became a quiet and phenomenal best seller, with thirty-five editions and the sale of some 88,000 copies between its initial publication and 1905. On his release from jail, Truelove was honored by his colleagues with much deserved praise and a purse of about two hundred pounds. He lived to see his ninetieth birthday.

### ROBERT WALLACE (1697–1771)

Wallace, a Scottish clergyman, was the author of *Various Prospects of Mankind, Nature and Providence,* published in London in 1761. He anticipated Malthus by a generation when he wrote there could not be a utopian or a "perfect government" because "mankind would increase so prodigiously that the earth would at last be overstocked, and become unable to support its numerous inhabitants." Godwin and Malthus were aware of Wallace's book.

### Charles Watts (1836–1906)

Watts was the son of a Wesleyan minister and younger brother of John Watts (1834–1866). Printer of the weekly *National Reformer* (1863–1866), Charles was secretary of Bradlaugh's National Secular Society (1866–1871) and sub-editor of the *National Reformer* from 1866 to 1871. But he broke with Bradlaugh on the question of the publication of Knowlton's book. Knowlton's work had been published in England (without any police, judicial, or other official interference) for nearly forty-three years by James Watson, Austin Holyoake, and Charles Watts. Watts pleaded guilty when prosecuted and thereby angered Bradlaugh, who came on the scene with Annie Besant. Some secularists did not want to be embroiled with Neo-Malthusian issues. Watts emigrated to Canada in 1866 but returned to England in 1891. He was the father of Charles Albert Watts, the publisher.

### James Watson (1799–1874)

An English freethought printer and publisher, Watson was one of the successors of Carlile in the struggle for freedom of the press. In 1832 he published the English edition of Owen's *Moral Physiology*. He also published, in 1834, the first British edition of Knowlton's *Fruits of Philosophy*. Watson took an active part in the radical movements for social and political reform of his day.

# BIBLIOGRAPHY

Arnstein, Walter L., *The Bradlaugh Case* (Oxford: Clarendon Press, 1965).

Ashton, T. S., *The Industrial Revolution, 1760–1830* (London: Oxford University Press, 1948).

*Autobiography of Mr. Bradlaugh: A Page of his Life* (London: Watts, 1873).

Banks, J. A., *Prosperity and Parenthood: A Study of Family Planning Among the Victorian Middle Class* (London: Routledge and Kegan Paul, 1954).

Banks, J. A. and Olive Banks, *Feminism and Family Planning in Victorian England* (Liverpool: Liverpool University Press, 1964).

Besant, Annie, *Autobiographical Sketches* (London: Freethought Publishing Co., 1885).

———, *Selection of Social and Political Pamphlets* (New York: Augustus M. Kelly, 1970).

———, *Charles Bradlaugh: A Character Sketch* (rpt. Madras: The Theosophical Publishing House, 1941).

———, *An Autobiography* (London: T. Fisher Unwin, 1893).

———, *Henry Varley Exposed* (London, 1881).

———, *The Law of Population: Its Consequences, and Its Bearing upon Human Conduct and Morals* (London: 1877).

Besterman, Theodore, *Mrs. Annie Besant: A Modern Prophet* (London: Routledge, 1934).

Bonar, James, *Malthus and His Work* (New York: Macmillan, 1933).

Bonner, Hypatia B., *Charles Bradlaugh: A Record of His Life and Work . . . with an Account of His Parliamentary Struggle, Politics and Teachings by John M. Robertson* (London, 1894).

———, *Charles Bradlaugh* (London: Unwin, 1894), 2 vols.

Bonner, Hypatia Bradlaugh and J. M. Robertson, *Charles Bradlaugh, His Life and Work* (London, 1898), 2 vols. Fifth edition (London: Fisher Unwin, 1902).

Bradlaugh, Charles, *The True Story of My Parliamentary Struggle* (London: Freethought Publishing Co., 1882).

——, *Jesus, Shelley and Malthus* (London, 1861).

Breed, Mary and Edith How-Martyn, *The Birth Control Movement in England* (London: John Bales, Sons and Danielson, 1930).

Carlile, Richard, *Every Woman's Book; or What is Love? Containing Most Important Instructions for the Prudent Regulation of the Principle of Love and the Number of a Family* (London: R. Carlile, 1828).

Chandrasekhar, S., *Infant Mortality, Population Growth and Family Planning in India*, 2nd ed. (London: Allen and Unwin; Chapel Hill: The University of North Carolina Press, 1975).

——, *Abortion in a Crowded World: The Problem of Abortion with Special Reference to India* (London: Allen and Unwin; Seattle: The University of Washington Press, 1974).

Clark, A., *History of the Diabolical Hand Bill, for Checking Population; with the various correspondence which has taken place, on this subject . . . with Observations* (Manchester, 1823).

Cohen, Chapman, *Bradlaugh and Ingersoll: A Centenary Appreciation of Two Great Reformers* (London: Pioneer Press, 1933).

Condorcet, Marie Jean Antoine Nicolas de Caritat, Marquis de, *Esquisse d'un tableau historique des progrès de l'esprit humain* (Paris, 1793).

Courtney, Janet Elizabeth, *Freethinkers of the Nineteenth Century* (Freeport, N.Y.: Books for Librarians Press, 1967).

Cox, Peter R., *Demography* (Cambridge: The University Press, 1950).

[Drysdale, George], a Graduate of Medicine, *Elements of Social Science* (London, 1859).

[——], *Physical, Sexual and Natural Religion*, by a Student of Medicine (London, 1854). Later editions were entitled *The Elements of Social Science.*

Elderton, Ethel M., *Report on the English Birthrate, Part 1, England North of Humber* (London: University of London, 1914).

Everseley, D. R. C., *Social Theories of Fertility and the Malthusian Debate* (London: Oxford University Press, 1959).

Field, James Alfred, *Essays on Population and Other Papers* (Chicago: University of Chicago Press, 1931).

Franklin, Benjamin, *Observations Concerning the Increase of Mankind and the Peopling of Countries, etc.* (Pennsylvania, 1751).

Fryer, Peter, *The Birth Controllers* (London: Corgi Books, 1967).

Glass, D. V., ed., *Introduction to Malthus* (London: Watts, 1953).

———, *Population Policies and Movements in Europe* (Oxford: Clarendon Press, 1940).

Godwin, William, *An Enquiry Concerning Political Justice and Its Influence on Morals and Happiness* (London, 1793).

Gray, Alexander, *The Socialist Tradition: Moses to Lenin* (London: Longmans Green, 1946).

Hazlitt, William, *A Reply to the Essay on Population by the Rev. T. R. Malthus. In a Series of Letters. To Which Are Added Extracts from the "Essay" with Notes* (London, 1807).

Himes, Norman E., *Medical History of Contraception* (1936; rpt. New York: Schocken Books, 1970).

———, ed., *Illustrations and Proofs of the Principle of Population by Francis Place;* being the first work on population in the English language recommending birth control, now exactly reproduced, with an introduction demonstrating Francis Place as the founder of the modern birth control movement, together with unpublished letters of Place on birth control, Coleridge's criticisms of Malthus' views on birth control. Critical and textual notes by Norman E. Himes (London: G. Allen and Unwin, 1930).

*In the High Court of Justice: Queen's Bench Division, June 18th, 1877: The Queen v. Charles Bradlaugh and Annie Besant* (London: Freethought Publishing Company, [1877]).

Knowlton, Charles, "Two Remarkable Lectures Delivered in Boston by Dr. C. Knowlton on the day of his leaving the Jail at East Cambridge, March 31, 1833, where he had been imprisoned, for publishing a book" (Boston: A. Kneeland, 1833).

*Law Reports, Queen's Bench Division, II*, 1876–77, XL, Victoria, "The Queen v. Charles Bradlaugh and Annie Besant," 28 June 1877 (London: William Clowes & Sons, 1877).

*Law Reports, Queen's Bench Division, III*, 1877–78, XLI, Victoria. In the Court of Appeal, 12 February 1878. "Charles Bradlaugh and Annie Besant v. the Queen" (London: William Clowes & Sons, [1878]).

Ledbetter, Rosanna, *A History of the Malthusian League, 1877–1927* (Columbus: Ohio State University Press, 1976).

Leybourne, Grace G. and Kenneth White, *Education and the Birth-Rate: A Social Dilemma* (London: Allen and Unwin, 1940).

Malthus, T. R., *An Essay on the Principle of Population as It Affects the Future Improvement of Society with Remarks on the Specula-tions of Mr. Godwin, M. Condorcet, and Other Writers* (London, 1798). Bonar's Edition, (London, 1926).

———, *An Essay on the Principle of Population; or, A View of Its Past and Present Effects on Human Happiness, with an Inquiry into Our Prospects Respecting the Future Removal or Mitigation of the Evils Which it Occasions.* A New Edition, very much en-larged (London, 1806).

McCleary, G. F., *Peopling the British Commonwealth* (London: Faber and Faber, 1955).

———, *The Malthusian Population Theory* (London: Faber and Faber, 1953).

———, *Population: Today's Question* (London: Allen and Unwin, 1938).

Meek, Ronald L., ed., *Marx and Engels on Malthus* (London: Law-rence and Wishart, 1954).

National Birth-Rate Commission, *The Declining Birth-Rate: Its Causes and Effects.* Report of and the chief evidence taken by the National Birth-Rate Commission, instituted with official recogni-tion, by the National Council of Public Morals—for the Promotion of Race Regeneration—Spiritual, Moral and Physical (London: Chapman and Hall, 1916).

Nethercot, Arthur E., *The First Five Lives of Annie Besant* (Chicago: University of Chicago Press, 1960).

———, *The Last Four Lives of Annie Besant* (Chicago: University of Chicago Press, 1963).

O'Hair, Madalyn Murray, *Champion of Liberty: Charles Bradlaugh* (New York: Arno Press and the New York Times, 1972).

Oser, Jacob, *Must Men Starve?* (London: Jonathan Cape, 1956).

Owen, Robert Dale, *Moral Physiology, or a Brief and Plain Treatise on the Population Question* (London: E. Truelove, 1832).

Pearsall, Ronald, *The Worm in the Bud. The World of Victorian Sex-uality* (London: Weidenfeld and Nicolson, 1969).

PEP, *Population Policy in Great Britain* (London: George Allen and Unwin, 1948).

Petersen, William, *Malthus* (Cambridge, Mass.: Harvard University Press, 1979).

———, *Population* (New York: Macmillan, 1975).

———, *The Politics of Population* (Garden City, N.Y.: Doubleday, 1964).

Prakasa, Sri, *Annie Besant as Woman and as Leader* (Bombay: Bharatiya Vidya Bhavan, 1962).

Quedalla, Philip, *The Queen and Mr. Gladstone* (London: Hodder, 1933), 2 vols.

*Queen v. Charles Bradlaugh and Annie Besant* (London: Freethought Publishing Company, 1878).

Reed, James, *From Private Vice to Public Virtue: The Birth Control Movement and American Society* (New York: Basic Books, 1978).

Royle, Edward, ed., *The Infidel Tradition: From Paine to Bradlaugh* (London: Macmillan, 1976).

Russell, Bertrand, and Patricia Russell, eds., *The Amberley Papers: The Letters and Diaries of Lord and Lady Amberley* (London: George Allen and Unwin, 1937), 2 vols.

Smith, Kenneth, *The Malthusian Controversy* (London: Routledge and Kegan Paul, 1951).

Stead, W. T., *Annie Besant: A Character Sketch* (Madras: The Theosophical Publishing House, 1941).

Talbot, Griffith G., *Population Problems of the Age of Malthus* (Cambridge: The University Press, 1926).

Thale, Mary, ed., *The Autobiography of Francis Place, 1771–1854* (London: Cambridge University Press, 1972).

Tribe, David H., *President Charles Bradlaugh, M.P.* (London: Elek, 1971).

United Kingdom, Royal Commission on Population, *Report* (London: H. M. Stationery Office, 1949), Cmd. 7695, Reprinted 1953.

Wallace, Robert, *A Dissertation on the Numbers of Mankind in Ancient and Modern Times* (Edinburgh, 1753).

———, *Various Prospects of Mankind, Nature and Providence* (London, 1761).

Wallas, Graham, *The Life of Francis Place* (New York: Knopf, 1918).

Webb, Beatrice, *My Apprenticeship* (London: Longmans, 1926).

Webb, Sidney, *The Decline in the Birth Rate,* Fabian Tract No. 131 (London: The Fabian Society, 1907).

West, Geoffrey [Wells, Geoffrey Harry], *Mrs. Annie Besant* (London: Gerald Howe, 1927).

Williams, Gertrude Leavenworth, *The Passionate Pilgrim: A Life of Annie Besant* (New York: Coward-McCann, 1931).

Williams, Gertrude Marvin, *Priestess of the Occult: Madame Blavatsky* (New York: Alfred Knopf, 1946).

*The Texts*

# FRUITS OF PHILOSOPHY.

## An Essay

ON THE

## POPULATION QUESTION.

By CHARLES KNOWLTON, M.D.

*" Author of Modern Materialism."*

SECOND NEW EDITION, WITH NOTES.

*ONE HUNDREDTH THOUSAND.*

LONDON :

FREETHOUGHT PUBLISHING COMPANY,

28, STONECUTTER STREET, E.C.

## PUBLISHERS' PREFACE

THE pamphlet which we now present to the public is one which has been lately prosecuted under Lord Campbell's Act, and which we republish in order to test the right of publication. It was originally written by Charles Knowlton, M.D., an American physician, whose degree entitles him to be heard with respect on a medical question. It is openly sold and widely circulated in America at the present time. It was first published in England, about forty years ago, by James Watson, the gallant Radical who came to London and took up Richard Carlile's work when Carlile was in jail. He sold it unchallenged for many years, approved it, and recommended it. It was printed and published by Messrs. Holyoake and Co., and found its place, with other works of a similar character, in their "Freethought Directory" of 1853, and was thus identified with Freethought literature at the then leading Freethought *depôt*. Mr. Austin Holyoake, working in conjunction with Mr. Bradlaugh at the *National Reformer* office, Johnson's Court, printed and published it in his turn, and this well-known Freethought advocate, in his "Large or Small Families," selected this pamphlet, together with R. D. Owen's "Moral Physiology" and the "Elements of Social Science," for special recommendation. Mr. Charles Watts, succeeding to Mr. Austin Holyoake's business, continued the sale, and when Mr. Watson died in 1875, he bought the plates of the work (with others) from Mrs. Watson, and continued to advertise and to sell it until December 23, 1876. For the last forty years the book has thus been identified with Freethought, advertised by leading Freethinkers, published under the sanction of their names, and sold in the head-quarters of Freethought literature. If during this long period the party has thus—without one word of protest—

circulated an indecent work, the less we talk about Freethought morality the better; the work has been largely sold, and if leading Freethinkers have sold it—profiting by the sale—in mere carelessness, few words could be strong enough to brand the indifference which thus scattered obscenity broadcast over the land. The pamphlet has been withdrawn from circulation in consequence of the prosecution instituted against Mr. Charles Watts, but the question of its legality or illegality has not been tried; a plea of "Guilty" was put in by the publisher, and the book, therefore, was not examined, nor was any judgment passed upon it; no jury registered a verdict, and the judge stated that he had not read the work.

We republish this pamphlet, honestly believing that on all questions affecting the happiness of the people whether they be theological, political, or social, fullest right of free discussion ought to be maintained at all hazards. We do not personally endorse all that Dr. Knowlton says: his "Philosophical Proem" seems to us full of philosophical mistakes, and—as we are neither of us doctors—we are not prepared to endorse his medical views; but since progress can only be made through discussion, and no discussion is possible where differing opinions are suppressed, we claim the right to publish all opinions, so that the public, enabled to see all sides of a question, may have the materials for forming a sound judgment.

The alterations made are very slight; the book was badly printed, and errors of spelling and a few clumsy grammatical expressions have been corrected: the subtitle has been changed, and in one case four lines have been omitted, because they are repeated word for word further on. We have, however, made some additions to the pamphlet, which are in all cases kept distinct from the original text. Physiology has made great strides during the past forty years, and not considering it right to circulate erroneous physiology, we submitted the pamphlet to a doctor in whose accurate knowledge we have the fullest confidence, and who is widely known in all parts of the world as the author of the "Elements of Social Science;" the notes signed "G. R."

are written by this gentleman.* References to other works are given in foot-notes for the assistance of the reader, if he desires to study the subject further.

Old Radicals will remember that Richard Carlile published a work entitled "Every Woman's Book," which deals with the same subject, and advocates the same object, as Dr. Knowlton's pamphlet. R. D. Owen objected to the "style and tone" of Carlile's "Every Woman's Book" as not being "in good taste," and he wrote his "Moral Physiology," to do in America what Carlile's work was intended to do in England. This work of Carlile's was stigmatised as "indecent" and "immoral," because it advocated, as does Dr. Knowlton's, the use of preventive checks to population. In striving to carry on Carlile's work, we cannot expect to escape Carlile's reproach, but whether applauded or condemned we mean to carry it on, socially as well as politically and theologically.

We believe, with the Rev. Mr. Malthus, that population has a tendency to increase faster than the means of existence, and that *some* checks must therefore exercise control over population; the checks now exercised are semistarvation and preventible disease; the enormous mortality among the infants of the poor is one of the checks which now keeps down the population. The checks that ought to control population are scientific, and it is these which we advocate. We think it more moral to prevent the conception of children, than, after they are born, to murder them by want of food, air, and clothing. We advocate scientific checks to population, because, so long as poor men have large families, pauperism is a necessity, and from pauperism grow crime and disease. The wage which would support the parents and two or three children in comfort and decency is utterly insufficient to maintain a family of twelve or fourteen, and we consider it a crime to bring into the world human beings doomed to misery or

[*G. R. (George Rex, a nickname) stands for Dr. George Drysdale (1825–1904), Scottish physician, ardent Neo-Malthusian, author of a popular and long-selling tome of the period, *The Elements of Social Science; the Physical, Sexual and Natural Religion* (1887). S. C.]

to premature death. It is not only the hard-working classes which are concerned in this question. The poor curate, the struggling man of business, the young professional man, are often made wretched for life by their inordinately large families, and their years are passed in one long battle to live; meanwhile the woman's health is sacrificed and her life embittered from the same cause. To all of these, we point the way of relief and of happiness; for the sake of these we publish what others fear to issue, and we do it, confident that if we fail the first time, we shall succeed at last, and that the English public will not permit the authorities to stifle a discussion of the most important social question which can influence a nation's welfare.

CHARLES BRADLAUGH
ANNIE BESANT

## PREFACE TO SECOND NEW EDITION

WE WERE not aware, when we published the first edition, that the editions published by James Watson, and professing to be reprinted by Holyoake and Co., Austin and Co., F. Farrah, J. Brooks, and Charles Watts, contained any variations. These variations are all of the most unimportant character, but as it was the edition issued by Mr. Watts, which was prosecuted, and as on careful reading we find there are some slight differences, the present edition is reprinted from his, with the exception of errors in printing and grammar.

CHARLES BRADLAUGH
ANNIE BESANT

## PREFACE

IT IS a notorious fact that the families of the married often increase beyond what a regard for the young beings coming into existence, or the happiness of those who gave them birth, would dictate; and philanthropists, of first-rate moral character, in different parts of the world, have for years been endeavouring to obtain and disseminate a knowledge of means whereby men and women may refrain at will from becoming parents, without even a partial sacrifice of the pleasure which attends the gratification of their productive instinct. But no satisfactory means of fulfilling this object were discovered until the subject received the attention of a physician, who had devoted years to the investigation of the most recondite phenomena of the human system, as well as to chemistry. The idea occurred to him of destroying the fecundating property of the sperm by chemical agents; and upon this principle he devised "checks," which reason alone would convince us must be effectual, and which have been proved to be so by actual experience.

This work, besides conveying a knowledge of these and other checks, treats of Generation, Sterility, Impotency, &c. &c. It is written in plain, yet chaste style. The great utility of such a work as this, especially to the poor, is ample apology, if apology be needed, for its publication.

# PHILOSOPHICAL PROEM

CONSCIOUSNESS is not a "principle" or substance of any kind; nor is it, strictly speaking, a property of any substance or being. It is a peculiar action of the nervous system; and the nervous system is said to be sensible, or to possess the property of sensibility, because those sentient actions which constitute our different consciousnesses, may be excited in it. The nervous system includes not only the brain and spinal marrow, but numerous soft white cords, called nerves, which extend from the brain and spinal marrow to every part of the body in which a sensation can be excited.

A sensation is a sentient action of a nerve and the brain; a thought or idea (both the same thing) is a sentient action of the brain alone. A sensation, or a thought, is consciousness, and there is no consciousness but that which consists either in a sensation or a thought.

Agreeable consciousness constitutes what we call happiness, and disagreeable consciousness constitutes misery. As sensations are a higher degree of consciousness than mere thoughts, it follows, that agreeable sensations constitute a more exquisite happiness than agreeable thoughts. That portion of happiness which consists in agreeable sensations is commonly called *pleasure*. No thoughts are agreeable except those which were originally excited by, or have been associated with, agreeable sensations. Hence if a person never had experienced any agreeable sensations, he could have no agreeable thoughts; and would of course be an entire stranger to happiness.

There are five species of sensation, seeing, hearing, smelling, tasting, and feeling. There are many varieties of feeling—as the feeling of hunger, thirst, cold, hardness, &c. Many of these feelings are excited by agents that act upon the exterior of the body, such as solid substances of every kind, heat, and various chemical irritants. Other feelings owe their existence to states or conditions of internal organs. These latter feelings are called *passions*.

Those passions which owe their existence chiefly to the state of the brain, or to causes acting directly upon the brain, are called the moral passions. They are grief, anger, love, &c. They consist of sentient actions which commence in the brain and extend to the nerves in the region of the stomach, heart, &c. But when the cause of the internal feeling or passion is seated in some organ remote from the brain, as in the stomach, the genital organs, &c., the sentient action which constitutes the passion, commences in the nerves of such organ, and extends to the brain; and the passion is called an *appetite, instinct* or *desire.* Some of these passions are natural, as hunger, thirst, the reproductive instinct, the desire to urinate, &c. Others are gradually acquired by habit. A *hankering* for stimulants, as spirits, opium and tobacco, is one of these.

Such is the nature of things that our most vivid and agreeable sensations cannot be excited under all circumstances, nor beyond a certain extent under any circumstances, without giving rise, in one way or another, to an amount of disagreeable consciousness, or misery, exceeding the amount of agreeable consciousness, which attend such ill-timed or excessive gratification. To excite agreeable sensations to a degree not exceeding this certain extent, is temperance; to excite them beyond this extent, is intemperance; not to excite them at all is mortification or abstinence. This certain extent varies with different individuals, according to their several circumstances, so that what would be temperance in one person may be intemperance in another.

To be free from disagreeable consciousness, is to be in a state which compared with a state of misery, is a happy state; yet absolute happiness does not consist in the absence of misery—if it do, rocks are happy. It consists, as aforesaid, in agreeable consciousness. That which enables a person to excite or maintain agreeable consciousness, is not happiness; but the *idea* of having such in one's possession is agreeable, and of course is a portion of happiness. Health and wealth go far in enabling a person to excite and maintain agreeable consciousness.

That which gives rise to agreeable consciousness is *good,* and we desire it. If we use it intemperately, such use is bad, but the thing itself is still good. Those acts (and intentions are acts of that part of man which intends) of human beings which tend to the promotion of happiness are good; but they are also called *virtuous,* to distinguish them from other things of the same tendency. There is nothing for the word *virtue* to signify but virtuous actions. Sin signifies nothing but sinful actions: and sinful, wicked, vicious, or bad actions, are those which are productive of more misery than happiness.

When an individual gratifies any of his instincts in a *temperate* degree, he adds an item to the sum total of human happiness, and causes the amount of human happiness to exceed the amount of misery, farther than if he had not enjoyed himself, therefore it is virtuous, or, to say the least, it is not vicious or sinful for him so to do. But it must ever be remembered, that this temperate degree depends on circumstances—that one person's health, pecuniary circumstances, or social relations may be such that it would cause more misery than happiness for him to do an act which, being done by a person under different circumstances, would cause more happiness than misery. Therefore it would be right for the latter to perform such act, but not for the former.

Again. Owing to his *ignorance,* a man may not be able to gratify a desire without causing misery (wherefore it would be wrong for him to do it), but with knowledge of means to prevent this misery, he may so gratify it that more pleasure than pain will be the result of the act, in which case the act to say the least is justifiable. Now, therefore, it is virtuous, nay, it is the *duty* for him who has a knowledge of such means, to convey it to those who have it not; for, by so doing, he furthers the cause of human happiness.

Man by nature is endowed with the talent of devising means to remedy or prevent the evils that are liable to arise from gratifying our appetites; and it is as much the duty of the physician to inform mankind of the means of preventing the evils that are liable to arise from gratifying the reproductive instinct, as it is to inform them how to keep clear of the gout or the dyspepsia. Let not the cold ascetic say we ought not to gratify our appetites any farther than is necessary to maintain health, and to perpetuate the species. Mankind will not so abstain, and if means to prevent the evils that may arise from a farther gratification can be devised, they *need not.* Heaven has not only given us the capacity of greater enjoyment, but the talent of devising means to prevent the evils that are liable to arise therefrom; and it becomes us, "with thanksgiving, to make the most of them."

*Showing how desirable it is, both in a political and a social point of view, for mankind to be able to limit, at will, the number of their offspring, without sacrificing the pleasure that attends the gratification of the reproductive instinct*

FIRST.—*In a political point of view.*—If population be not restrained by some great physical calamity, such as we have reason to hope will not hereafter be visited upon the children of men, or by some *moral restraint,* the time will come when the earth cannot support its inhabitants. Population, unrestrained, will double three times in a century. Hence, computing the present population of the earth at 1,000 millions, there would be at the end of the 100 years from the present time, 8,000 millions.

> At the end of 200 years   64,000 millions.
> At the end of 300 years  512,000 millions.

And so on, multiplying by eight for every additional hundred years. So that in 500 years from the present time, there would be thirty-two thousand seven-hundred and sixty-eight times as many inhabitants as at present. If the natural increase should go on without check for 1,500 years, one single pair would increase to more than *thirty-five thousand one hundred and eighty-four* times as many as the present population of the whole earth!

Some check, then, there must be, or the time will come when millions will be born but to suffer and to perish for the necessaries of life. To what an inconceivable amount of human misery would such a state of things give rise! And must we say that vice, war, pestilence, and famine are desirable to prevent it? Must the friends of temperance and domestic happiness stay their efforts? Must peace societies excite to war and bloodshed? Must the physician cease to investigate the nature of contagion, and to search for the means of destroying its baneful influence? Must he that becomes diseased be marked as a victim to die for the public good, without the privilege of making an effort to restore him to health? And in case of a failure of crops in one part of the world, must the other parts withhold the means of supporting life, that the far greater evil of excessive population throughout the globe may be prevented? Can there be no effectual moral restraint, attended with far less human misery than such physical calamities as these? Most surely there can. But what is it? Malthus, an English writer on the subject of population, gives us none but celibacy to a late age. But how foolish it is to suppose that men and women will become as monks and nuns during the very holiday of their existence, and abjure during the fairest years of life the nearest and dearest of social relations, to avert a catastrophe, which they, and perhaps their children, will not live to witness. But, besides being ineffectual, or if effectual, requiring a great sacrifice of enjoyment, this restraint is highly objectionable on the score of its demoralising tendency. It would give rise to a frightful increase of prostitution, of intemperance and onanism, and prove destructive to health and moral feelings. In spite of preaching, human nature will ever remain the same; and that restraint which forbids the gratification of the reproductive instinct, will avail but little with the mass of mankind. The checks to be hereafter mentioned, are the only moral restraints to population known to the writer, that are unattended with serious objections.

Besides starvation with all its accompanying evils, overpopulation is attended with other public evils, of which may be mentioned ignorance and slavery. Where the mass of the people must toil incessantly to obtain support, they must remain ignorant; and where ignorance prevails tyranny reigns.*

*The Scientific part of Malthus's Doctrine of Population is not very clearly or correctly given in the above passages. His great theory, now so generally held by the most eminent political economists, is that the increase of population is always powerfully checked in old countries by the difficulty of increasing the supply of food; that the existing evils of poverty and low wages are really at bottom caused by this check, and are brought about by

Second.—*In a social point of view.*—"Is it not notorious that the families of the married often increase beyond what a regard for the young beings coming into the world, or the happiness of those who give them birth, would dictate? In how many instances does the hard-working father, and more especially the mother, of a poor family remain slaves throughout their lives, tugging at the oar of incessant labour, toiling to live, and living but to toil; when, if their offspring had been limited to two or three only, they might have enjoyed comfort and comparative affluence? How often is the health of the mother, giving birth every year to an infant—happy if it be not twins—and compelled to toil on, even at those times when nature imperiously calls for some relief from daily drudgery—how often is the mother's comfort, health, nay, even her life thus sacrificed? Or if care and toil have weighed down the spirit, and at length broken the health of the father, how often is the widow left, unable, with the most virtuous intentions, to save her fatherless offspring from becoming degraded objects of charity, or profligate votaries of vice!

"Nor is this all. Many women are so constituted that they cannot give birth to healthy—sometimes not to living children. Is it desirable—is it moral, that such women should become pregnant? Yet this is continually the case. Others there are, who ought never to become parents; because, if they do, it is only to transmit to their offspring grievous hereditary diseases, which render such offspring mere subjects of misery throughout their sickly existence. Yet such women will not lead a life of celibacy. They marry. They become parents, and the sum of human misery is increased by their doing so. But it is folly to expect that we can induce such persons to live the lives of Shakers. Nor is it

the pressure of population on the soil, and the continual overstocking of the labour markets with labourers; and hence that the only way in which Society can escape from poverty, with all its miseries, is by putting a strong restraint on their great natural powers of multiplication. "It is not in the nature of things," he says, "that any permanent and general improvement in the condition of the poor can be effected without an increase in the preventive check to population."—G. R.

necessary;—all that duty requires of them is to refrain from becoming parents. Who can estimate the beneficial effect which a rational moral restraint may thus have on the health and beauty, and physical improvement of our race throughout future generations."

Let us now turn our attention to the case of unmarried youth.

"Almost all young persons, on reaching the age of maturity, desire to marry. That heart must be very cold, or very isolated, that does not find some object on which to bestow its affections. Thus, early marriages would be almost universal did not prudential considerations interfere. The young man thinks 'I cannot marry yet, I cannot support a family. I must make money first and think of a matrimonial settlement afterwards.'

"And so he goes to making money, fully and sincerely resolved, in a few years to share it with her whom he now loves. But passions are strong and temptations great. Curiosity perhaps introduces him into the company of those poor creatures whom society first reduces to a dependence on the most miserable of mercenary trades, and then curses for being what she has made them. There his health and moral feelings alike make shipwreck. The affections he had thought to treasure up for their first object are chilled by dissipation and blunted by excess. He scarcely retains a passion but avarice. Years pass on—years of profligacy and speculation—and his first wish is accomplished, his fortune is made. Where now are the feelings and resolves of his youth.

'Like the dew on the mountain,
Like the foam on the river,
Like the bubble on the fountain,
They are gone—and for ever.'

"He is a man of pleasure, a man of the world. He laughs at the romance of his youth, and marries a fortune. If gaudy equipage and gay parties confer happiness he is happy. But if they be only the sunshine on the stormy sea below, he is a victim to that system of morality which forbids a reputable connection until the period when provision has been made for a large expected family. Had he married the first object of his choice, and simply delayed becoming a father until his prospects seemed to warrant it, how different might have been his lot. Until men and women are absolved from the fear of becoming parents, except when they themselves desire it, they ever will form mercenary and demoralizing connections, and seek in dissipation the happiness they might have found in domestic life.

"I know that this, however common, is not a universal case. Sometimes the heavy responsibilities of a family are incurred at all risks; and who shall say how often a life of unremitting toil and poverty is the consequence? Sometimes, if even rarely, the young mind does hold to its first resolves. The youth plods through years of cold celibacy and solitary anxiety, happy, if before the best hours of his life are gone, and its warmest feelings withered, he may return to claim the reward of his forbearance and his industry. But even in this comparatively happy case, shall we count for nothing the years of ascetic sacrifice at which after happiness is purchased? The days of youth are not too many, nor its affections too lasting. We may, indeed, if a great object require it, sacrifice the one and mortify the other. But is this, in itself, desirable? Does not wisdom tell us that such a sacrifice is a dead loss—to the warm-hearted often a grievous one? Does not wisdom bid us temperately enjoy the springtime of life, 'while the evil day come not, nor the years draw nigh, when we shall say we have no pleasure in them.'

"Let us say, then, if we will, that the youth who thus sacrifices the present for the future, chooses wisely between the two evils, profligacy and asceticism. This is true. But let us not imagine the lesser evil to be a good. It is *not* good for man to be alone. It is for no man or woman's happiness or benefit that they should be condemned to Shakerism. It is a violence done to the feelings and an injury to the character. A life of rigid celibacy, though infinitely preferable to a life of dissipation, is yet fraught with many evils. Peevishness, restlessness, vague longings, and instability of character, are amongst the least of these. The mind is unsettled and the judgment warped. Even the very instinct which is thus mortified assumes an undue importance, and occupies a portion of the thoughts which does not of right or nature belong to it, and which during a life of satisfied affection it would not obtain."

In many instances the genital organs are rendered so irritable by the repletion to which unnatural continency gives rise, and by much thinking, caused by such repletion, as to induce a disease known to medical men by the name of *Gonorrhœa Dormientium.* It consists in an emission or discharge of the semen during sleep. This discharge is immediately excited in most instances by a lascivious dream, but such dream is caused by the repletion and irritability of the genital organs. It is truly astonishing to what a degree of mental anguish the disease gives rise in young men. They do not understand the nature, or rather, the cause of it. They think it depends on a weakness—indeed the disease is often called a 'seminal weakness'—and that the least gratification in a natural way would but serve to increase it. Their anxiety about it weakens the whole system. This weakness they erroneously attribute to the discharges, they think themselves totally disqualified for entering into or enjoying the married state. Finally, the genital and mental organs act and react upon each other so perniciously, as to cause a degree of nervousness, debility, emaciation, and melancholy—in a word a wretchedness that sets description at defiance. Nothing is so effectual in curing this diseased state of body and mind in young men as marriage. All restraint, fear, and solicitude should be removed.

"Inasmuch, then as the scruples of incurring heavy responsibilities deter from forming moral connections, and encourage intemperance and prostitution, the knowledge which enables man to limit the number of his offspring, would in the present state of things save much unhappiness and prevent many crimes. Young persons sincerely attached to each other and who might wish to marry, would marry early; merely resolving not to become parents until prudence permitted it. The young man, instead of solitary toil and vulgar dissipation, would enjoy the society and the assistance of her he had chosen as his companion; and the best years of life, whose pleasures never return, would not be squandered in riot, nor lost through mortification."*

*The passages are quoted from Robert Dale Owen's "Moral Physiology." (Published by E. Truelove.)—[Publishers' note.]

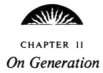

CHAPTER II
## *On Generation*

I HOLD the following to be important and undeniable truths: That every man has a natural right both to receive and convey a knowledge of all the facts and discoveries of every art and science, excepting such only as may be secured to some particular person or persons by copyright or patent. That a physical truth in its general effect cannot be a moral evil. That no fact in physics or in morals ought to be concealed from the enquiring mind.

Some may make a misuse of knowledge, but that is their fault, and it is not right that one person should be deprived of knowledge, of spirits, of razors, or of anything else which is harmless in itself and may be useful to him, because another may misuse it.

The subject of generation is not only interesting as a branch of science, but it is so connected with the happiness of mankind that it is highly important in a practical point of view. Such, to be sure, is the custom of the age that it is not considered a proper subject to investigate before a popular assembly, nor is it proper to attend the calls of nature in a like place, yet they must and ought to be attended to, for the good—the happiness of mankind require it; so too, for like reason the subject of generation ought to be investigated until it be rightly understood by all people, but at such opportunities as the good sense of every individual will easily decide to be proper. This I presume to say, not simply upon the abstract principle that all knowledge of nature's workings is useful, and the want of it disadvantageous, but from the known moral fact, that ignorance of this process has in many instances proved the cause of a lamentable "mishap," and more especially as it is essential to the attainment of the great advantages which it is the chief object of this work to bestow upon mankind.

People generally, as it was the case with physicians until late years, entertain a very erroneous idea of what takes place in the process of conception. Agreeably to this idea, the "check" which I consider far preferable to any other would not be effectual, as would be obvious to all. Consequently, entertaining this idea, people would not have due confidence in it. Hence it is necessary to correct a long held and widely extended error. But this I cannot expect to do by simply saying it is an error. Deeply rooted and hitherto undisputed opinions are not so easily eradicated. If I would convince any one that the steps in one of the most recondite processes of nature are not such as he has always believed, it will greatly serve my purpose to show what these steps are. I must first prepare him to be reasoned with, and then reason the matter all over with him—I must point out the facts which disprove his opinion, and show that my own is unattended with difficulties.

But what can be more obvious than that it is absolutely impossible to explain any process or function of the animal economy so as to be understood, before the names of the organs which perform this function have been defined, that is, before the organs themselves have been described. Now it is well known to every anatomist, and indeed it must be obvious to all, that in describing any organ or system of organs we must always begin with some external and known part, and proceed regularly, step by step, to the internal and unknown. As in arithmetic, "everything must be understood as you go along."

Fully to effect the objects of this work, it is, therefore, a matter of necessity that I give an anatomical description of certain parts—even external parts—which some, but for what I have just said, might think it useless to mention. It is not to gratify the idle curiosity of the light-minded that this book is written, it is for *utility* in the broad and truly philosophical sense of the term: nay, farther, it shall, with the exception of here and there a little spicing,* be confined to *practical utility*. I shall therefore endeavour to treat of the subject in this chapter so as to be under-

*This is an Americanism, which appears to us to convey a false idea. If it refers to the cases used as illustrations, Dr. Knowlton is more sparing in his use of them than either Dr. Bull or Dr. Chavasse.—[Publishers' note.]

stood, without giving any description of the male organs of generation; though I hold it an accomplishment for one to be able to speak of those organs, as diseases often put them under the necessity of doing, without being compelled to use low and vulgar language. But I must briefly describe the female organs; in doing which, I must, of course, speak as do other anatomists and physiologists; and whoever objects to this will discover more affectation and prudery than good sense and goodwill to mankind.

The adipose, or fatty matter, immediately over the share bone, forms a considerable prominence in females, which, at the age of puberty, is covered with hair, as in males. This prominence is called Mons Veneris.

The exterior orifice commences immediately below this. On each side of this orifice is a prominence continued from the mons veneris, which is largest above and gradually diminishes as it descends. These two prominences are called the Labia Externa, or external lips. Near the latter end of pregnancy they become somewhat enlarged and relaxed, so that they sustain little or no injury during parturition. Just within the upper or anterior commissure formed by the junction of these lips, a little round oblong body is situated. The body is called the clitoris. Most of its length is bound down, as it were, pretty closely to the bone: and it is of very variable size in different females. Instances have occurred where it was so enlarged as to enable the female to have venereal commerce with others; and in Paris this fact was once made a public exhibition of to the medical faculty. Women thus formed appear to partake in their general form of the male character, and are termed hermaphrodites. The idea of human beings, called hermaphrodites, which could be either father or mother, is, doubtless, erroneous. The clitoris is analogous in its structure to the penis, and like it, is exquisitely sensible, being, as it is supposed, the principal seat of pleasure. It is subject to erection or distension, like the penis, from like causes.

The skin which lines the internal surface of the external lips is folded in such a manner as to form two flat bodies, the exterior edges of which are convex. They are called the nymphae. They extend downward, one on each side, from the clitoris to near the middle of the external orifice, somewhat diverging from each other. Their use is not very evident. The orifice of the urethra (the canal, short in females, which leads to the bladder) is situated an inch or more farther inward than the clitoris, and is a little protuberant.

Passing by the external lips, the clitoris, the nymphae, and the orifice of the urethra, we come to the membrane called the hymen. It is situated just at or a trifle behind the orifice of the urethra. It is stretched across the passage, and were it a complete septum, it would close up the anterior extremity of that portion of the passage which is called the vagina. But the instances in which the septum or partition is complete, are very rare; there being, in almost all cases, an aperture either in its centre, or, more frequently in its anterior edge, giving the membrane the form of a crescent. Through this aperture passes the menstrual fluid. Sometimes, however, this septum is complete, and the menstrual fluid is retained month after month, until appearances and symptoms much like those of pregnancy are produced, giving rise perhaps to unjust suspicions. Such cases require the simple operation of dividing the hymen. In many instances the hymen is very imperfect, insomuch that some have doubted whether it is to be found in the generality of virgins. Where it exists, it is generally ruptured in the first intercourse of the sexes, and the female is said to lose her virginity. In some rare instances it is so very strong as not to be ruptured by such intercourse, and the nature of the difficulty not being understood, the husband has sued for a divorce. But everything may be put to rights by a slight surgical operation. The parts here described are among those called the external parts of generation.

The internal organs of generation consist, in the female, of the Vagina, the Uterus, the Ovaries and their appendages.

The Vagina is a membranous canal commencing at the hymen, and extending to the uterus. It is a little curved, and extends backwards and upwards between the bladder, which lies before and above it, and that extreme portion of the bowels called the rectum, which lies behind it. The coat or membrane which lines the internal surface of the vagina forms a number of transverse ridges. These ridges are to be found only in the lower or anterior half of the vagina, and they do not extend all round the vagina, but are situated on its anterior and posterior sides, while their lateral sides are smooth. I mention these ridges because a knowledge of them may lead to a more effectual use of one of the checks to be made known hereafter.

The Uterus, or womb, is also situated between the bladder and the rectum, but above the vagina. Such is its shape that it has been compared to a pear with a long neck. There is, of course, considerable difference between the body and the neck, the first being twice as broad as the last. Each of these parts is somewhat flattened. In subjects of mature age, who have never been pregnant, the whole of the uterus is about two inches and a half in length, and more than an inch and a half in breadth at the broadest part of the body. It is near an inch in thickness. The neck of the uterus is situated downwards, and may be said to be inserted into the upper extremity of the vagina. It extends down into the vagina the better part of an inch. In the uterus is a cavity which approaches the triangular form, and from which a canal passes down through the neck of the uterus into the vagina. This cavity is so small that its sides are almost in contact. So that the uterus is a thick, firm organ for so small a one. Comparing the cavity of the uterus to a triangle, we say the upper side or line of this triangle is transverse with respect to the body, and the other two lines pass downwards and inwards, so that they would form an angle below, did they not before they meet take a turn more directly downwards to form the canal just mentioned. In each of the upper angles there is an orifice of such size as to admit of a hog's bristle. These little orifices are the mouths of two tubes, called the fallopian tubes, of which more will be said presently. The canal which passes through the neck of the uterus, connecting the cavity of this organ with that of the vagina, is about a quarter of an inch in diameter. It is different from other ducts, for it seems to be a part of the cavity from which it extends, inasmuch as when the cavity of the uterus is enlarged in the progress of pregnancy, this canal is gradually converted into a part of that cavity.

The lower extremity of the neck of the uterus is irregularly convex and tumid. The orifice of the canal in it is oval, and so situated that it divides the convex surface of the lower extremity of the neck in two portions, which are called the lips of the uterus. The anterior is thicker than the posterior. The orifice itself is called *os tincœ* or *os uteri,* or in English, the mouth of the womb. When the parts are in a weak, relaxed state, the mouth or neck of the uterus is quite low, and in almost all cases it may be reached by a finger introduced into the vagina, especially by a second person who carries the hand behind.

The Ovaries are two bodies of a flattened or oval form, one of which is situated on each side of the uterus at a little distance from it, and about as high up as where the uterus becomes narrow to form its neck. The longest diameter of the ovarium is about an inch. Each ovarium has a firm coat of membrane. In those who have not been pregnant, it contains from ten to twenty *vesicles,* which are little round bodies, formed of a delicate membrane, and filled with a transparent fluid. Some of these vesicles are situated so near the surface of the ovarium as to be prominent on its surface. They are of different sizes, the largest nearly a quarter of an inch in diameter.*

In those in whom conception has ever taken place, some of these vesicles are removed, and in their place a cicatrix or scar is formed which continues through life. However, the number of cicatrices does not always correspond with the number of conceptions. They often exceed it, and are sometimes found where conception has not been known to take place.

The Fallopian Tubes are two canals four or five inches in length, proceeding from the upper angles of the cavity of the

*The vesicles here mentioned are the so-called Graafian vesicles, or ovisacs, each of which contains in its interior a little ovum or egg. In the human female the ovum is extremely minute, so as only to be visible with the aid of a lens. The Graafian vesicles are not limited to a certain small number, as was formerly thought, but continue to be formed in the ovaries, and to discharge at intervals mature ova during the whole of the fruitful period of life.—G. R.

uterus, in a transverse direction in respect to the body. Having so proceeded for some distance, they turn downwards towards the ovaries. At their commencement in the uterus they are very small, but they enlarge as much as they progress. The large ends which hang loose, terminate in open mouths, the margins of which consist of fimbriated processes, and nearly touch the ovaria.

We are now prepared to treat of conception. Yet, as menstruation is closely connected with it, and as a knowledge of many things concerning menstruation may contribute much to the well being of females, for whom this work is at least as much designed as for males, I shall first briefly treat of this subject.

*Menstruation.*—When females arrive at the age of puberty they begin to have a discharge once every month, by way of the vagina, of the colour of blood. This discharge is termed the menses. To have it, is to menstruate. The age at which menstruation commences varies with different individuals, and also in different climates. The warmer the climate the earlier it commences and ceases. In temperate climates it generally commences at the age of fourteen or fifteen, and ceases at forty-four, or a little later.* Whenever it commences the girl acquires a more womanly appearance. It is a secretion of the uterus, or in other words, the minute vessels distributed to the inner coat of the uterus, select as it were, from the blood, and pour out in a gradual manner the materials of this fluid. It has one of the properties, colour, of blood, but it does not coagulate, or separate into different parts like blood, and cannot properly be called blood.† When this discharge is in all respects regular, it amounts in most females to six

---

*Dr. Chavasse, on p. 94 of his "Advice to a Wife" (published by W. H. Smith & Son), gives instances of very early menstruation and consequent fecundity.—[Publishers' note.]

†"The menstrual discharge," says Dr. Kirks, "consists of blood effused from the inner surface of the uterus, and mixed with mucus from the uterus, vagina, and external parts of the generative apparatus. Being diluted by this admixture, the menstrual blood coagulates less perfectly than ordinary blood; and the frequent acidity of the vaginal mucus tends still further to diminish its coagulability."—"Handbook of Physiology," 8th ed., p. 727, 1874.—G. R.

or eight ounces, and is from two to four days' continuance. During its continuance the woman is said to be unwell, or out of order. Various unpleasant feelings are liable to attend it; but when it is attended with severe pain, as it not unfrequently is, it becomes a disease, and the woman is not likely to conceive until it be cured. During the existence of the "turns," or "monthlies," as they are often called, indigestible food, dancing in warm rooms, sudden exposure to cold or wet, and mental agitations should be avoided as much as possible. The "turns" do not continue during pregnancy, nor nursing, unless nursing be continued too long. The milk becomes bad if nursing be continued after the "turns" recommence. Some women, it is true, are subject to a slight hemorrhage that sometimes occurs with considerable regularity during pregnancy, and which has led them to suppose they have their turns at such terms; but it is not so; the discharge at such times is real blood.*

The use of the menstrual discharge seems to be, to prepare the uterine system for conception. For females do not become pregnant before they commence, nor after they cease having their turns; nor while they are suppressed by some disease, by cold or by nursing. Some credible women, however, have said that they become pregnant while nursing, without having had any turn since their last lying-in. It is believed that in these cases they had some discharge, colourless perhaps, which they did not notice, but which answered the purposes of the common one. Women are not nearly so likely to conceive during the week before a monthly, as during the week immediately after.† But although the use of this secretion seems to be to prepare for conception, it is not to be inferred that the reproductive instinct ceases at the "turn of life," or when the woman ceases to menstruate. On the contrary, it is said that this passion often increases at this period, and continues in a greater or less degree to an extreme age.

*Consult on the whole of this Dr. Chavasse's book, pp. 91–101, where full details are given.—[Publishers' note.]

†See, however, Dr. Bull's "Hints to Mothers," pp. 51–58, and 127–129 (published by Longmans, Green & Co.)—[Publishers' note.]

*Conception.*—The part performed by the male in the reproduction of the species consists in exciting the orgasm of the
female, and depositing the semen in the vagina. Before I inquire
what takes place in the females, I propose to speak of the semen.

This fluid, which is secreted by the testicles, may be said to
possess three kinds of properties, physical, chemical, physiological. Its physical properties are known to every one—it is a thick-
ish, nearly opaque fluid, of a peculiar odour, saltish taste, &c. As
to its chemical properties, it is found by analysis to consist of 900
parts of water, 60 of animal mucilage, 10 of soda, 30 of phos-
phate of lime. Its physiological property is that of exciting the
female genital organs in a peculiar manner.

When the semen is examined by a microscope, there can be
distinguished a multitude of small animalculae, which appear to
have a rounded head and a long tail. These animalculae move
with a certain degree of rapidity. They appear to avoid the light
and to delight in the shade. Leeuwenhoek, if not the discoverer
of the seminal animalculae, was the first who brought the fact of
their existence fully before the public. With respect to their size,
he remarked that ten thousand of them might exist in a space
not larger than a grain of sand. They have a definite figure, and
are obviously different from the animalculae found in any other
fluid.* Leeuwenhoek believed them to be the beginnings of future animals—that they are of different sexes, and even thought
he could discover a difference of sex, upon which depends the
future sex of the foetus. Be this as it may, it appears to be admitted on all hands that the animalculae are present in the semen of
the various species of male animals, and that they cannot be
detected when either from age or disease the animals are rendered sterile. "Hence," says Bostock, "we can scarcely refuse
our assent to the position, that these animalculae are in some
way or other instrumental to the production of the foetus." The
secretion of the semen commences at the age of puberty. Before
this period the testicles secrete a viscid, transparent fluid, which

*See Dr. Carpenter's "Animal Physiology," p. 558 (published by H. G.
Bohn); Nichol's "Human Physiology," pp. 253–255 (published by Trubner
& Co.)—[Publishers' note.]

has never been analysed, but which is doubtless essentially different from semen. The revolution which the whole economy undergoes at this period, such as the tone of the voice, the development of hairs, the beard, the increase of the muscles and bones, &c., is intimately connected with the existence of the testicles and the secretion of this fluid.* "Eunuchs preserve the same form as in childhood; their voice is effeminate, they have no beard, their disposition is generally timid; and finally their physical and moral character very nearly resembles that of females. Nevertheless, many of them take delight in venereal intercourse, and give themselves up with ardour to a connexion which must always be unfruitful"†

The part performed by the female in the reproduction of the species is far more complicated than that performed by the male. It consists, in the first instance, in providing a substance, which, in connection with the male secretion, is to constitute the foetus; in furnishing a suitable situation in which the foetus may be developed; in affording due nourishment for its growth; in bringing it forth, and afterwards furnishing it with food especially adapted to the digestive organs of the young animal. Some parts of this process are not well understood, and such a variety of hypotheses have been proposed to explain them, that Drelincourt, who lived in the latter part of the 17th century, is said to have collected 260 hypotheses of generation.

It ought to be known that women have conceived when the semen was merely applied to the parts anterior to the hymen, as the internal surface of the external lips, the nymphae, &c. This is proved by the fact that several cases of pregnancy have occurred when the hymen was entire. This fact need not surprise us; for, agreeable to the theory of absorption, we have to account for it only to suppose that some of the absorbent vessels are situated anterior to the hymen—a supposition by no means unreasonable.

There are two peculiarities of the human species respecting

*Nichol's "Human Physiology," pp. 255, 256.—[Publishers note.]
†Magendie's Physiology.—[Author's note.]

conception, which I will notice. First, unlike other animals, they are liable—and for what has been proved to the contrary, equally liable—to conceive at all seasons of the year. Second, a woman rarely, if ever, conceives until after having had several sexual connections; nor does one connection in fifty cause conception in the matrimonial state, where the husband and wife live together uninterruptedly. Public women rarely conceive, owing probably to a weakened state of the genital system, induced by too frequent and promiscuous intercourse.

It is universally agreed, that some time after a fruitful connection, a vesicle (two in case of twins) of one or the other ovary becomes so enlarged that it bursts forth from the ovary and takes the name of ovum; which is taken up, or rather received, as it bursts forth, by the fimbriated extremity of the fallopian tube, and is then slowly conducted along the tube into the uterus to the inner surface of which it attaches itself.* Here it becomes developed into a full-grown foetus, and is brought forth about forty-two weeks from the time of conception by a process termed

*Since Dr. Knowlton's work was written, the very important fact has been discovered that ova are periodically discharged from the ovaries in the human female and other animals, not in consequence of fruitful connection having taken place, as was formerly believed, but quite independently of intercourse with the male. Such a discharge of ova occurs in the lower animals at the time of heat or rut, and in women during menstruation. At each menstrual period, a Graafian vesicle becomes enlarged, bursts, and lets the ovum which it contains escape into the Fallopian tube, along which it passes to the uterus. "It has long been known," says Dr. Kirke, "that in the so-called oviparous animals, the separation of ova from the ovary may take place independently of impregnation by the male, or even of sexual union. And it is now established that a like maturation and discharge of ova, independently of coition, occurs in Mammalia, the periods at which the matured ova are separated form the ovaries and received into the Fallopian tubes being indicated in the lower Mammalia by the phenomena of *heat* or *rut;* in the human female by the phenomena of *menstruation.* Sexual desire manifests itself in the human female to a greater degree at these periods, and in the female of mammiferous animals at no other time. If the union of the sexes takes place, the ovum may be fecundated, and if no union occur it perishes. From what has been said, it may, therefore, be concluded that the two states, heat and menstruation, are analogous, and that the essential accompaniment of both is the maturation and extrusion of ova."—"Handbook of Physiology," p. 724.—G. R.

parturition. But one grand question is, how the semen operates in causing the vesicle to enlarge, etc; whether the semen itself or any part thereof reaches the ovary, and if so, in what way it is conveyed to them. It was long the opinion that the semen was ejected into the uterus in the act of coition, and that it afterwards by some unknown means found its way into and along the fallopian tubes to the ovary. But there are several facts which weigh heavily against this opinion, and some that entirely forbid it. In the first place, there are several well-attested instances in which impregnation took place while the hymen remained entire; where the vagina terminated in the rectum, and where it was so contracted by a cicatrix as not to admit the penis. In all these cases the semen could not have been lodged anywhere near the mouth of the uterus, much less ejected into it. Secondly, it has followed a connection where, from some defect in the male organs, as the urethra terminating some inches behind the end of the penis, it is clear that the semen could not have been injected into the uterus, nor even near its mouth. Third, the neck of the unimpregnated uterus is so narrow as merely to admit a probe, and is filled with a thick tenacious fluid, which seemingly could not be forced away by any force which the male organ possesses of ejecting the semen, even if the mouth of the male urethra were in opposition with that of the uterus. But, fourth, the mouth of the uterus is by no means fixed. By various causes it is made to assume various situations, and probably the mouth of the urethra rarely comes in contact with it.

Fifth. "The tenacity of the male semen is such as renders its passage through the small aperture in the neck of the uterus impossible, even by a power or force much superior to that which we may rationally suppose to reside in the male organs of generation.

Sixth. "Harvey and De Graaf dissected animals at almost every period after coition, for the express purpose of discovering the semen, but were never able to detect the smallest vestige of it in the uterus in any one instance.*

*Dewees' Essay on Superfoetation.—[Author's note.]

Aware of the insurmountable objections to this view of the manner in which the semen reaches the ovary, it has been supposed by some physiologists that the semen is absorbed from the vagina into the great circulating system, where it is mixed, of course, with the blood, and goes the whole round of the circulation, subject to the influence of those causes which produce great changes in the latter fluid.

To this hypothesis it may be objected, that while there is no direct evidence in support of it, it is exceedingly unreasonable, inasmuch as we can scarcely believe that the semen can go the whole round of circulation, and then find its way to the ovary in such a pure unaltered state as the experiments of Spallanzani prove it must be in, that it may impregnate.

A third set of theorists have maintained that an imperceptible something, which they have called *aura seminalis,* passes from the semen lodged in the vagina to the ovary, and excites those actions which are essential to the development of an ovum. Others, again, have told us, that it is all done by sympathy. That neither the semen nor any volatile part of it finds its way to the ovary; but that the semen excites the parts with which it is in contact in a peculiar manner, and by a law of the animal economy, termed sympathy or consent of parts, a peculiar action commences in the ovary, by which an ovum is developed, &c."

To both these conjectures it may be objected, that they have no other foundation but the supposed necessity of adopting them, to account for the effect of impregnation; and further, they "make no provision for the formation of mules; for the peculiarities of, and likeness to, parents, and for the propagation of predisposition to disease, from parent to child; for the production of mulattoes, &c.

A fifth, and, to me, far more satisfactory view of the subject than any other, is that advanced by our distinguished countryman, Dr. Dewees, of Philadelphia. It appears to harmonize with all known facts relating to the subject of conception; and something from analogy may also be drawn in its favour. It is this: that there is a set of absorbent vessels leading directly from the inner surface of the *labia externa* and the vagina to the ovaries, the whole office of which vessels is, to absorb the semen and convey it to the ovaries.* I do not know that these vessels have yet been fully discovered; but in a note on the sixteenth page of his "Essays on Various Subjects," the doctor says: "The existence of these vessels is now rendered almost certain, as Dr. Gartner, of Copenhagen, has discovered a duct leading from the ovary to the vagina."

Another question of considerable moment relating to generation is, from which parent are the first rudiments of the foetus derived.

The earliest hypothesis with which we are acquainted, and which has received the support of some of the most eminent of the moderns, ascribes the original formation of the foetus to the combination of particles of matter derived from each of the parents. This hypothesis naturally presents itself to the mind as the obvious method of explaining the necessity for the co-operation of the two sexes, and the resemblance in external form, and even in mind and character, which the offspring frequently bears to the male parent. "The principal objections," says Bostock, "to this hypothesis, independent of the want of any direct proof of a female seminal fluid, are of two descriptions, those which depend upon the supposed impossibility of unorganised matter forming

*This view is not held at the present day. The commonly received doctrine now is that the seminal fluid enters the uterus, whether during the intercourse or after it, and passes along the Fallopian tubes to the ovaries; and that fecundation takes place at some point of this course, most frequently in the tubes, but also at times in the ovary itself, or even, perhaps, in the uterus. It is essentially necessary for fecundation that the spermatozoa should come into actual contact with the ovum. "That the spermatozoa make their way towards the ovarium, and fecundate the ovum either before it entirely quits the ovisac or very shortly afterwards," says Dr. Carpenter, "appears to be the general rule in regard to the Mammalia; and their power of movement must obviously be both vigorous and long continued to enable them to traverse so great an extent of mucus membrane, especially when it is remembered that they ascend in opposition to the direction of the ciliary movement of the epithetial cells, and to the downward peristaltic action of the Fallopian tubes. . . . There can be no doubt that it is in the contact of the spermatozoa with the ovum, and in the changes which occur as the immediate consequence of that contact, that the act of fecundation essentially consists."—"Principles of Human Physiology," 8th ed., p. 961, 1876.—G. R.

an organised being, and those which are derived from observations and experiments of Haller and Spallanzani, which they brought forward in support of their theory of pre-existent germs."

In relation to these objections I remark, first, that those whose experience has been with hale females, I suspect can have no doubt but that the female orgasm increases like that of the male, until an emission of fluid of some kind or other takes place. But whether this secretion may properly be called semen, whether any part of it unites with the male semen in forming the rudiments of the foetus, is another question. For my part I am inclined to the opinion that it does not.* I rather regard it as the result of exalted excitation, analogous to the increased secretion of other organs from increased stimulation; and if it be for any object or use, as it probably is, it is that of affording nature a means of relieving herself; or, in other words, of quieting the venereal passion. If this passion, being once roused, could not by some means or other be calmed, it would command by far too great a proportion of our thoughts, and with many constitutions, the individuals, whether male or female, could not conduct themselves with due decorum. One fact which leads me to think that the female secretion in the act of coition is not essential to impregnation, is, that many females have conceived, if their unbiassed testimony may be relied on, when they experienced no pleasure. In these cases it is more than probable that there was no orgasm, nor any secretion or emission of fluid on the part of the female.

As to the objection of the supposed impossibility of unorganised matter forming an organised being, I do not conceive that it weighs at all against the hypothesis before us, for I do not believe such a thing takes place, even if we admit that "the original formation of the foetus is a combination of particles of mat-

*With regard to this secretion in the female, which has nothing of a seminal character, Dr. Carpenter observes, "Its admixture with the male semen has been supposed to have some connection with impregnation; but no proof whatever has been given that any such admixture is necessary."—"Human Physiology," p. 961.—G. R.

ter derived from each of the parents." What do, or rather what ought we to mean by organised matter? Not, surely, that it exhibits some obvious physical structure, unlike what is to be found in inorganic matter, but that it exhibits phenomena, and of course may be said to possess properties unlike any kind of inorganic matter. Matter unites with matter in three ways, mechanically, chemically, and organically, and each mode of union gives rise to properties peculiar to itself. When matter unites organically, the substance or being so formed exhibits some phenomena essentially different from what inorganic bodies exhibit. It is on this account that we ascribe to organic bodies certain properties, which we call physiological properties, such as contractility, sensibility, life, &c. When, from any cause, these bodies have undergone such a change that they no longer exhibit the phenomena peculiar to them, they are said to have lost these properties, and to be dead. A substance need not possess all the physiological properties of an animal of the higher orders, to entitle it to the name of an organised or living substance, nor need it possess the physical property of solidity. The blood, as well as many of the secretions, does several things, exhibits several phenomena, which no mechanical or mere chemical combinations of matter do exhibit. We must therefore ascribe to it certain physiological properties, and regard it as an organised, a living fluid, as was contended by the celebrated John Hunter. So with respect to the semen, it certainly possesses physiological properties, one in particular, peculiar to itself, namely, the property of impregnating the female; and upon no sound principle can it be regarded in any other light than as an organised, and of course a living fluid. And if the female secretion or any part of it unite with the male secretion in the formation of the rudiments of the foetus in a different manner than any other substance would, then it certainly has the property of doing so, whether we give this property a name or not; and a regard to the soundest principles of physiology compels us to class this property with the physiological or vital, and of course to regard this secretion as an organised and living fluid. So, then, unorganised matter does not form an organised being, admitting the hypothesis before us as correct.

That organised beings should give rise to other organised beings under favourable circumstances as to nourishment, warmth, &c., is no more wonderful than that fire should give rise to fire when air and fuel are present. To be sure, there are some minute steps in the process which are not fully known to us; still, if they ever should be known, we should unquestionably see that there is a natural cause for every one of them; and that they are all consonant with certain laws of the animal economy. We should see no necessity of attempting to explain the process of generation by bringing to our aid, or rather to the darkening of the subject, any imaginary principle, as the *nisus formativus* of Blumenbach.

As to the "observations and experiments of Haller and Spallanzani," I think with Dr. Bostock that they weigh but little, if any, against the theory before us. I shall not be at the labour of bringing them forward, and shewing their futility as objections to this theory, for I am far from insisting on the correctness of it; that is, I do not insist that any part of the female secretion, during coition, unites with the male semen in the formation of the rudiments of the foetus.

The second hypothesis or theory I shall notice, as to the rudiments of the foetus, is that of Leeuwenhoek, who regarded the seminal animalcules of the male semen as the proper rudiments of the foetus, and thinks that the office of the female is to afford them a suitable receptacle, where they may be supported and nourished until they are able to exist by the exercise of their own functions. This is essentially the view of the subject which I adopt, and which I intend to give more particularly presently.

I know of no serious objections to this hypothesis; nothing but the "extreme improbability," as its opponents say, "that these animalculae should be the rudiments of being so totally dissimilar to them." But I wish to know if there is more difference between a foetus and a seminal animalcule, than there is between a foetus and a few material particles in some other form than that of such animalcule?

The third hypothesis, or that of pre-existing germs, proceeds upon a precisely opposite view of the subject to that of Leeuwenhoek, namely, that the foetus is properly the production of the female; that it exists previous to sexual congress, with all its organs, in some part of the uterine system; and that it receives no proper addition from the male, but that the seminal fluid acts merely by exciting the powers of the foetus, or endowing it with vitality.

It is not known who first proposed this hypothesis; but, strange as it may appear, it has had the support of such names as Bonnet, Haller, and Spallanzani, and met with a favourable reception in the middle of the last century. Agreeable to this hypothesis, our common mother, Eve, contained a number of homuncules (little men) one within another, like a nest of boxes, and all within her ovaries, equal to all the number of births that have ever been, or ever will be, not to reckon abortions! Were I to bring forward all the facts and arguments that have been advanced in support of this idea, it seems to me I should fail to convince sound minds of its correctness; as to arguments against it, they surely seem uncalled for. Having now presented several hypotheses of generation, some as to the manner in which the semen reaches or influences the ovary, and others as to the rudiments of the foetus, I shall now bring together those views which upon the whole appear to me the most satisfactory.

I believe with Dr. Dewees that a set of absorbent vessels extend from the innermost surface of the *labia externa*, and from the vagina to the ovary, the whole office of which is to take up the semen or some part thereof and convey it to the ovary. I believe with Leeuwenhoek, that the seminal animalcules are the proper rudiments of the foetus, and are perhaps of different sexes, that in case of impregnation one of them is carried not only to, but into a vesicle of an ovary, which is in a condition to receive, and be duly affected by it.* It is here surrounded by the

---

*The opinion that the spermatozoa or seminal filaments are real animalcules is now abandoned, but it is held by Dr. Carpenter and other authorities that they do actually, as here stated, penetrate into the interior of the ovum. "The nature of impregnation," says Dr. Hermann, "is as yet unknown. In all probability it is, above all, essential, in order that it should occur, that one or more spermatozoa should penetrate the ovum. At any rate, spermatozoa have been found within the fecundated eggs of the most diverse species of animals."—"Elements of Human Physiology," translated from the 5th ed., by Dr. Gamgee, p. 534, 1875.—G. R.

122

albuminous fluid which the vesicle contains. This fluid being somewhat changed in its qualities by its new comer, stimulates the minute vessels of the parts which surround it, and thus causes more of this fluid to be formed, and while it affords the animalcule material for its development, it puts the delicate membrane of the ovary which retains it in its place upon the stretch, and finally bursts forth surrounded probably by an exceedingly delicate membrane of its own. This membrane with the albuminous fluid it contains, and the animalcule in the centre of it, constitutes the ovum or egg. It is received by the fimbriated extremity of the fallopian tube, which by this time has grasped the ovary, and is by this tube slowly conveyed into the uterus, to the inner surface of which it attaches itself, through the medium of the membrane, which is formed by the uterus itself in the interim, between impregnation and the arriving of the ovum in the way I have just mentioned.

The idea that a seminal animalcule enters an ovum while it remains in the ovary, was never before advanced to my knowledge; hence I consider it incumbent upon me to advance some reasons for the opinion.

First, it is admitted on all hands, that the seminal animalculae are essential to impregnation, since "they cannot be detected when either from age or disease the animal is rendered sterile."

Second, the ovum is impregnated while it remains in the ovary. True, those who have never met with Dr. Dewees' theory, and who, consequently have adopted the idea that the semen is ejected into the uterus, as the least improbable of any with which they were acquainted, have found it very difficult to dispose of the fact that the ovum is impregnated in the ovary, and have consequently presumed this is not generally the case. They admit it is certainly so sometimes, and that it is difficult to reject the conclusion that it is always so. Dr. Bostock—who doubtless had not met with Dewees' theory at the time he wrote, and who admits it impossible to conceive how the semen can find its way along the fallopian tubes—how it can find its way towards the ovary farther, at most, than into the uterus, and consequently cannot see how the ovum can be impregnated into the ovary— says: "Perhaps the most rational supposition may be that the ovum is transmitted to the uterus in the unimpregnated state; but there are certain facts which seem almost incompatible with this idea, especially the cases which not unfrequently occur of perfect foetuses having been found in the tubes, or where they escaped them into the cavity of the abdomen. Hence it is demonstrated that the ovum is occasionally impregnated in the tubes (why did he not say ovaria?), and we can scarcely resist the conclusion that it must always be the case." ᔕᔕᔕ "Haller discusses this hypothesis (Bostock's 'most natural supposition, perhaps,') and decides against it." ᔕᔕᔕ "The experiments of Cruikshank, which were very numerous, and appear to have been made with the requisite degree of skill and correctness, led to the conclusion that the rudiment of the young animal is perfected in the ovarium." ᔕᔕᔕ "A case is detailed by Dr. Granville, of a foetus which appears to have been lodged in the body of the ovarium itself, and it is considered by its author as a proof that conception always takes place in this organ." The above quotations are from the third volume of Bostock's Physiology.

Now as the seminal animalculae are essential to impregnation, and as the ovum is impregnated in the ovarium, what more probable conjecture can we form than an animalcule, as the real proper rudiment of the foetus, enters the ovum, where, being surrounded with albuminous fluid with which it is nourished, it gradually becomes developed? It may be noticed that Leeuwenhoek estimates that ten thousand animalculae of the human semen may exist in a space not larger than a grain of sand. There can, therefore, be no difficulty in admitting that they may find their way along exceedingly minute vessels from the vagina, not only to, but into the ovum, while situated in the ovarium.

I think no one can be disposed to maintain that the animalcule merely reaches the surface of the ovum,* and thus impregnates it. But possibly some may contend that its sole office is to stimulate the ovum, and in this way set going that train of actions which are essential to impregnation. But there is no evi-

*I say surface of the ovum, for it is probably not a mere drop of fluid, but fluid surrounded with an exceedingly delicate membrane.—[Author's note.]

dence in favour of this last idea, and certainly it does not so well harmonise with the fact that the offspring generally partakes more or less of the character of its male parent. As Dr. Dewees says of the doctrine of sympathy: "It makes no provision for the formation of mules; for the peculiarities of, and likeness to, parents; and for the propagation of predisposition to disease from parent to child; for the production of mulattoes, etc."

Considering it important to do away with the popular and mischievous error, that the semen must enter the uterus to effect impregnation, I shall, in addition to what has been already advanced, here notice the experiments of Dr. Haighton. He divided the fallopian tubes in numerous instances, and found that after this operation a foetus is never produced, but that *corpora lutea* were formed. The obvious conclusions from these facts are, that the semen does not traverse the fallopian tubes to reach the ovaria; yet that the ovum becomes impregnated while in the ovarium, and consequently that the semen reaches the ovarium in some way, except by the uterus and fallopian tubes. I may remark, however, that a *corpus luteum* is not positive proof that impregnation at some time or other has taken place; yet they are so rarely found in virgins that they were regarded as such proof until the time of Blumenbach, a writer of the present century.*

"Harvey and De Graaf dissected animals at almost every period after coition, for the express purpose of discovering the semen, but were never able to detect the smallest vestige of it in the uterus in any one instance."—*Dewees' Essay on Superfoetation.* The fact of superfoetation furnishes a very strong argument against the idea that the semen enters the uterus in impregnation.

A woman being impregnated while she is already impregnated constitutes superfoetation. It is established beyond a doubt

---

*A *corpus luteum* is a little yellowish body, formed in the ovary by changes that take place in the Graafian vesicle, after it has burst and discharged its contents. *Corpora lutea* were formerly considered a sure sign of impregnation, as they were thought to be developed only or chiefly in cases of pregnancy, but it is now known that they occur in all cases where a vesicle has been ruptured and an ovum discharged; though they attain a larger size and are longer visible in the ovary when pregnancy takes place than when it does not.—G. R.

that such instances have occurred, yet those who have supposed that it is necessary for the semen to pass through the mouth of the uterus to produce conception, have urged that superfoetation could not take place, because, say they—and they say correctly—"so soon as impregnation shall have taken place, the *os uteri* closes, and becomes impervious to the semen, ejected in subsequent acts of coition."

Dr. Dewees relates two cases, evidently cases of superfoetation, that occurred to his own personal knowledge. The first shows that, agreeable to the old theory, the semen must have met with other difficulties than a closed mouth of the uterus—it must have passed through several membranes, as well as the waters surrounding the foetus, to have reached even the uterine extremity of a fallopian tube. The second case I will give in his own words:—

"A white woman, servant to Mr. H., of Abington township, Montgomery county, was delivered about five and twenty years since of twins, one of which was perfectly white, the other perfectly black. When I resided in that neighborhood I was in the habit of seeing them almost daily, and also had frequent conversations with Mrs. H. respecting them. She was present at their birth, so that no possible deception could have been practised respecting them. The white girl is delicate, fair-skinned, light-haired, and blue-eyed, and is said very much to resemble the mother. The other has all the characteristic marks of the African; short of stature, flat, broad-nosed, thick-lipped, woolly-headed, flat-footed, and projecting heels; she is said to resemble a negro they had on the farm, but with whom the woman never would acknowledge an intimacy; but of this there was no doubt, as both he and the white man with whom her connection was detected, ran from the neighborhood so soon as it was known the girl was with child."

I am aware that some have thought they had actually discovered semen in the uterus, while Ruysch, an anatomist of considerable eminence, who flourished at the close of the 17th century, asserted in the most unequivocal manner, that he found the semen in its gross white state in one of the fallopian tubes of a woman, who died very soon after, or during the act of coition; but, says Dewees, "the semen, after it has escaped from the penis, quickly loses its albuminous appearance, and becomes as thin and transparent as water. And we are certain that Ruysch was mistaken. Some alteration in the natural secretion of the parts was mistaken for semen. This was nowise difficult for him to do, as he had a particular theory to support, and more especially as this supposed discovery made so much for it. It is not merely speculative when we say that some change in the natural secretion of the parts may be mistaken for semen; for we have the testimony of Morgagni on our side. He tells us he has seen similar appearances in several instances in virgins and others, who had been subject during their lives to leucorrhoea, and that it has been mistaken by some for male semen."

On the whole I would say, that in some instances, where the mouth of the uterus is uncommonly relaxed, the semen may, as it were, accidentally have found its way into it; but that is not generally the case, nor is it essential to impregnation; and further, that whatever semen may at any time be lodged in the uterus, has nothing to do with conception. It is not consistent with analogy to suppose that the uterus has vessels for absorbing the semen and conveying it to the ovaria, considering the other important functions which we know it performs.

The circumstances under which a female is most likely to conceive are, first, when she is in health; second, between the ages of twenty-six and thirty; third, after she has a season been deprived of those intercourses she had previously enjoyed; fourth, soon after menstruating. Respecting this latter circumstance, Dr. Dewees remarks, "Perhaps it is not erring greatly to say, that the woman is liable to conceive at any part of the menstrual interval. It is generally supposed, however, that the most favourable instant is, immediately after the catamenia have ceased;" perhaps this is so as a general rule, but it is certainly liable to exceptions,* and he relates the following case which occurred to his own notice:—

*This view, which concerns a question of the utmost practical importance, is held at the present day by the great majority of physiologists. It is

127

"The husband of a lady who was obliged to absent himself many months in consequence of the embarrassment of his affairs, returned one night clandestinely; his visit being only known to his wife, his mother, and myself. The consequence of this visit was the impregnation of his wife. The lady was at this time within a week of her menstrual period; and as this did not fail to take place, she was led to hope she had not suffered by the visit of her husband. But her catamenia not appearing at the next period, gave rise to a fear that she had not escaped; and the birth of a child nine months and thirteen days from the night of this clandestine visit, proved her apprehensions too well grounded."

I think this case is an exception to a general rule; and, furthermore, favours an idea which reason and a limited observation, rather than positive knowledge, has led me to advance above, namely, that a woman is more likely to conceive, other things being the same, after being deprived for a season of those intercourses she had previously enjoyed. Had this lady's husband remained constantly at home, she would probably either not have conceived at all, or have done so a fortnight sooner than she did.

---

believed that although conception may occur at other times, it is much more likely to happen from intercourse a few days before or after the menstrual periods; that is to say, during the time when ova are in process of being ripened and detached from the ovaries, and before they perish and are conveyed out of the body. "There is good reason to believe," says Dr. Carpenter, "that in the human female the sexual feeling becomes stronger at the period of menstruation; and it is quite certain that there is a greater aptitude for conception, immediately before and after that epoch, than there is at any intermediate period. This question has been made the subject of special inquiry by M. Raciborski, who affirms that the exceptions to the rule—that conception occurs immediately before or after, or during menstruation—are not more than 6 or 7 percent. Indeed, in his latest work on the subject, he gives the details of 15 cases, in which the date of conception could be accurately fixed, and the time of the last appearance of the catamenia was also known, and in all but one of them, the correspondence between the two periods was very close."—"Human Physiology," p. 959. So, too, Dr. Kirkes remarks, that "although conception is not confined to the periods of menstruation, yet it is more likely to occur within a few days after cessation of the menstrual flux than at other times."—"Handbook of Physiology," p. 725.

This case is also remarkable for two other facts; one "that a woman in perfect health, and pregnant with a healthy child, may exceed the period of nine months by several days; the other, that a check is not always immediately given to the catamenial flow, by an ovum being impregnated." Probably it is not so generally so as many suppose.

The term of utero-gestation, or the length of time from conception to the commencement of labour, is not precisely determined by physiologists. "It seems, however," says Dr. Dewees, "from the best calculations that can be made, that nine calendar months, or forty weeks, approaches the truth so nearly, that we can scarcely need desire more accuracy, could it be obtained." Unquestionably, however, some cases exceed this period by many days, or even weeks, and it has been a question much agitated, how far this period is ever exceeded. It is a question of some moment in a legal point of view. Cases are reported where the usual period was exceeded by five or six months; cases, too, where the circumstances attending them, and the respectability of their reporters are such as to command our belief. Dr. Dewees has paid much attention to this subject, and he declares himself entirely convinced, "that the commonly fixed period may be extended from thirteen days to six weeks, under the influence of certain causes or peculiarities of constitution."*

These occasional departures from the general rule, will, perhaps be the more readily admitted when we consider that they are not confined to the human species. From the experiments of Tessier it appears that the term of utero-gestation varies greatly with the cow, sheep, horse, swine, and other animals to which his attention was directed.

Properly connected with the subject of generation, are the signs of pregnancy. Dr. Dewees remarks that "our experience furnishes no certain mark by which the moment conception takes place is to be distinguished. All appeals by the women to particular sensations experienced at the instant should be very

*See tables in Dr. Bull's "Hints to Mothers," pp. 130–141.—[Publishers' note.]

guardedly received, for we are certain they cannot be relied upon; for enjoyment and indifference are alike fallacious. Nor are certain nervous tremblings, nausea, palpitation of the heart, the sensation of something flowing from them during coition, &c., more to be relied upon." Burns, however, says, "some women feel, immediately after conception, a peculiar sensation, which apprises them of their situation, but such instances are not frequent, and generally the first circumstances which lead a woman to suppose herself pregnant, are the suppression of the menses;" a fickle appetite, some sickness, perhaps vomiting, especially in the morning; returning qualms, or langour in the afternoon; she is liable to heartburn, and to disturbed sleep. The breasts at first often become smaller, sometimes tender; but about the third month they enlarge, and occasionally become painful. The nipple is surrounded with an areola or circle of a brown colour, or at least of a colour sensibly deeper or darker than before. She loses her looks, becomes paler, and the under part of the lower eyelid is often somewhat of a leaden hue. The features become sharper, and sometimes the whole body begins to emaciate, while the pulse quickens. In many instances particular sympathies take place, causing salivation, toothache, jaundice, &c. In other cases very little disturbance is produced, and the woman is not certain of her condition until the time of quickening, which is generally about four months from conception. It is possible for women to mistake the effects of wind for the motion of the child, especially if they have never borne children, and be anxious for a family; but the sensation produced by wind in the bowels is not confined to one spot, but is often felt at a part of the abdomen where the motion of a child could not possibly be felt. Quite as frequently, perhaps, do fleshy women think themselves dropsical, and mistake motions of the child for movements of water within the abdominal cavity. The motion of the child is not to be confounded with the sensation sometimes produced by the uterus rising out of the pelvis, which produces the feeling of fluttering. At the end of the fourth month the uterus becomes so large that it is obliged to rise out of the pelvis, and if this elevation takes place suddenly, the sensation accompanying it is pretty strong, and the woman at the time feels sick or faint, and in irritable habits, even a hysterical fit may accompany it. After this the morning sickness and other sympathetic effects of pregnancy generally abate, and the health improves.

Very soon after impregnation, if blood be drawn, and suffered to stand a short time undisturbed, it will become sizy, of a yellowish or blueish colour, and somewhat of an oily appearance. But we cannot from such appearances of the blood alone pronounce a woman pregnant, for a suppression of the menses, accompanied with a febrile state, may give the blood a like appearance as pregnancy, so also may some local disease. Of the above mentioned symptoms, perhaps there is no *one* on which we can place more reliance than the increased colour of the circle around the nipple.*

Six or eight weeks after conception, the most sure way of ascertaining pregnancy is to examine the mouth and neck of the uterus, by way of the vagina. The uterus will be found lower down than formerly, its mouth is not directed so much forward as before impregnation, it is more completely closed, and the neck is felt to be thicker, or increased in circumference. When raised on the finger it is found to be heavier or more resisting. Whoever makes this examination must have examined the same uterus in an unimpregnated state, and retained a tolerably correct idea of its feeling at that time, or he will be liable to uncertainty, because the uterus of one woman is naturally different in magnitude from that of another, and the uterus is frequently lower down than natural, from other causes than pregnancy.†

It has not been fully ascertained how long it is after a fruitful connection before any effect is produced upon the ovaria, that is, before any alteration could be discovered, were the female to be dissected. But Haighton's experiments have established the fact, that with rabbits, whose term of utero-gestation is but thirty days, no effect is propagated to the ovaria until nearly fifty hours after coition; we should judge, therefore, that with the human species it must be several days, and it is generally estimated by

*See "Advice to a Wife." P. H. Chavasse, pp. 115–124, where many details are given.—[Publishers' note.]

†No one but a doctor, or one trained in physiology, could, of course, make any such examination with safety and utility.—[Publishers' note.]

physiologists that the ovum does not reach the uterus until the expiration of twenty days from the time of connection.*

It is probable that in all cases in which any matter is absorbed from any part of the animal system, some little time is required for such matter, after its application, to stimulate and arouse the absorbent vessels to action; hence it is probable, that after the semen is lodged in the vagina, it is many minutes, possibly some hours, before any part of it is absorbed.

CHAPTER III

## Of Promoting and Checking Conception

STERILITY depends either on imperfect organisation, or imperfect action of the organs of generation. In the former cases, which are rare, the menses do not generally appear, the breasts are not developed, and the sexual desire is inconsiderable. There is no remedy in these cases.

The action may be imperfect in several respects. The menses may be obstructed or sparing, or they may be too profuse or frequent. It is extremely rare for a woman to conceive who does not menstruate regularly. Hence where this is the case the first step is to regulate this periodical discharge.† For this purpose the advice of a physician will generally be required, for these irregularities depend upon such various causes and require such variety of treatment, that it would be inconsistent with the plan of this work to attempt to give instructions for remedying them. A state of exhaustion, or weakness of the uterine system, occasioned by too frequent intercourse, is a frequent cause of sterility. The sterility of prostitutes is attributed to this cause, but I doubt it being the only one. With females who are apparently healthy,

*"The time occupied in the passage of the ovum, from the ovary to the uterus," says Dr. Kirkes, "occupies probably eight or ten days in the human female."—"Handbook of Physiology," p. 741.—G. R.

†Chavasse, pp. 87–107, deals very fully with this point.—[Publishers' note.]

the most frequent cause is a torpor, rather than weakness, of the genital organs.

For the removal of sterility from this cause, I shall give some instructions, and this I do the more readily because the requisite means are such as will also regulate the menses in many cases, where they do not appear so early in life, so freely or so frequently as they ought.

In the first place it will generally be necessary to do something towards invigorating the system by exercise in the open air, by nourishing food of easy digestion, by sufficient dress, particularly flannel, and especially by strict temperance in all things. With this view also, some scales which fall from the blacksmith's anvil, of some steel filings, may be put into old cider or wine (cider the best), and after standing a week or so, as much may be taken two or three times a day as can be borne without disturbing the stomach. All the while the bowels are to be kept rather open, by taking from one to three of *Pill rufi* every night on going to bed. These pills consist of four parts of aloes, two parts of myrrh, and one of saffron, by weight.

These measures having been regularly pursued until the system be brought into a vigorous state, medicines which are more particularly calculated to arouse the genital organs from a state of torpor may be commenced, and continued for months if necessary. The cheapest, most simple (and I am not prepared to say it is not the most effectual in many cases), is cayenne. All the virtues of this article are not generally known even to physicians. I know it does not have the effect upon the coats of the stomach that many have conjectured. It may be taken in the quantity of from one to two rising tea-spoonsful, or even more, every day, upon food or on any liquid vehicle. Another medicine of much efficacy is Dewees' Volatile Tincture of Guaiac. It is generally kept by apothecaries, and is prepared as follows:—

Take of Gum Guaiacum, in powder eight ounces; carbonate of Potash, or of Soda, or (what will answer) Salaeratus, three drachms; Allspice, in powder, two ounces; any common spirits of good strength, two pounds, or what is about the same, two pints and a gill. Put all into a bottle, which may be shaken now and then, and the use of it may be commenced in a few days. To every gill of this, at least a large tea-spoonful of Spirits of Ammonia is to be added. A tea-spoonful is to be taken for a dose, three times a day, in a glass of milk, cider, or wine. It is usually given before eating; but if it should chance to offend the stomach when taken before breakfast, it may in this case be taken an hour after.

Dr. Dewees found this tincture, taken perhaps for months, the most effectual remedy for painful menstruation, which is an obstinate complaint. If there be frequent strong pulse, heat, thirst, florid countenance, &c., it is not to be taken until these symptoms be removed by low diet, a few doses of salts, and bleeding, if required.

A third medicine for arousing the genital organs is tincture of Spanish Flies. But I doubt its being equal, in sterility, to the above-mentioned medicines, though it may exceed them in some cases, and may be tried if these fail. A drachm of them may be put to two gills of spirits. Dose, 25 drops, in water, three times a day, increasing each one by two or three drops, until some degree of stranguary occurs, then omit until this pass off, as it will in a day or two. Should the stranguary be severe, drink freely of milk and water, slippery elm, or flax seed tea.

In many cases of sterility, where the general health is considerably in fault, and especially where the digestive organs are torpid, I should have much confidence in a Thomsonian course. It is calculated to arouse the capillary vessels throughout the whole system, and thus to open the secretions, to remove obstructions, and free the blood of those effete and phlegmy materials which nature requires to be thrown off. The views of the Thomsonians as to heat and cold, appear to me unphilosophical. But this has nothing to do with the efficiency of their measures.

In relation to sterility, I would here bring to mind, what has been before stated, that a woman is most likely to conceive immediately after a menstrual turn. And now, also, let me suggest the idea that nature's delicate beginnings may be frustrated by the same means that put her agoing. This idea is certainly important when the woman is known to have miscarried a number of times. Sterility is sometimes to be attributed to the male, though he apparently be in perfect health. It would be an interesting fact to ascertain if there be no seminal animalcules in these cases; and whether medicines of any kind are available.

It has been ascertained that a male and female may be sterile in relation to each other, though neither of them be so with others.

The foregoing measures for sterility are also suitable in cases of impotency. This term, I believe, is generally confined to, and defined as, a want of desire or ability, or both, on the part of the male; but I see no good reason why it should not comprehend the cases in which there is neither desire nor pleasure with the female. Such females, it is true, may be fruitful; but so, on the other hand, the semen may not have lost its fecundating property. Impotency, at a young or middle age, and in some situations in life especially, is certainly a serious misfortune to say the least of it. The whole evil by no means consists in every case, in the loss of a source of pleasure. All young people ought to be apprised of the causes of it—causes which in many instances greatly lessen one's ability of giving and receiving that pleasure which is the root of domestic happiness. I shall allude to one cause, that of premature, and especially solitary gratification, in another place. Intemperance in the use of spirits is another powerful cause. Even a moderate use of spirits, and also of tobacco, in any form, have some effect. It is a law of the animal economy, that no one part of the system can be stimulated or excited, without an expense of vitality, as it is termed. That part which is stimulated draws the energy from other parts. And hence it is, that close and deep study, as well as all the mental passions when excessive, impair the venereal appetite. All excesses, all diseases and modes of life, which impair the general health, impair this appetite, but some things more directly and powerfully than others.

As to the remedies for impotency, they are much the same as for sterility. It is of the first importance that the mind be relieved from all care and anxiety. The general health is to be improved by temperance, proper exercise in the open air, cheerful company, change of scenery, or some occupation to divert the mind without requiring much exercise of it; nourishing food of easy digestion; flannel worn next to the skin. The cold bath may be tried, and if it be followed by agreeable feelings, it will do good. The bowels may be gently stimulated by the pills before mentioned; and the preparation of iron also, already mentioned, should be taken.

To stimulate the genital organs more directly, cayenne, Dewees' tincture of guaiac, or tincture of flies may be taken. I have given directions for making and taking the tincture of flies, chiefly because it is esteemed one of the best remedies for impotency caused by or connected with nocturnal emissions, to which I have before alluded.

It is in cases where little or no pleasure, nor erection attend these emissions—cases brought on by debauchery, or in elderly persons, that I would recommend tincture of flies, and the other measures above mentioned. In some bad cases, enormous doses of this tincture are required, say two or three hundred drops. Yet the best rule for taking it is that already given, namely, begin with small doses, and gradually increase until some stranguary be felt, or some benefit be received. In this affection, as well as in all cases of impaired virility, the means I have mentioned are to be pursued for a long time, unless relief be obtained. These have cured after having been taken for a year or more without the result. In all cases of impotency not evidently depending upon disease of some part besides the genital organs, I should have much confidence in blisters applied to the lower part of the spine.

Occasional nocturnal emissions, accompanied with erection, and pleasure, are by no means to be considered a disease; though they have given many a one much uneasiness. Even if they be frequent, and the system considerably debilitated, if not caused by debauch, and the person be young, marriage is the proper measure.

There have been several means proposed and practised for checking conception. I shall briefly notice them, though a knowledge of the best is what most concerns us. That of withdrawal immediately before emission is certainly effectual, if practised with sufficient care. But if (as I believe) Dr. Dewees' theory of conception be correct; and as Spallanzani's experiments show that only a trifle of semen even largely diluted with water, may impregnate by being injected into the vagina, it is clear that nothing short of entire withdrawal is to be depended upon. But the old notion that the semen must enter the uterus to cause conception, has led many to believe that a partial withdrawal is sufficient, and it is on this account that this error has proved mischievous, as all important errors generally do. It is said by those who speak from experience, that the practice of withdrawal has an effect upon the health similar to temperance in eating. As the subsequent exhaustion is probably mainly owing to the shock the nervous system sustains in the act of coition, this opinion may be correct. It is further said that this practice serves to keep alive those fine feelings with which married people first come together. Still I leave it for every one to decide for himself whether this check be so far satisfactory, as not to render some other very desirable.

As to the baudruche, which consists in a covering used by the male, made of very delicate skin, it is by no means calculated to come into general use. It has been used to secure from syphilitic affections.

Another check which the old idea of conception has led some to recommend with considerable confidence, consists in introducing into the vagina, previous to connexion, a very delicate piece of sponge, moistened with water, to be immediately afterwards withdrawn by means of a very narrow ribbon attached to it.* But as our views would lead us to expect, this check has not proved a sure preventative. As there are many little ridges or folds in the vagina, we cannot suppose the withdrawal of the sponge would dislodge all the semen in every instance. If, however, it were well moistened with some liquid which acted chemically upon the semen, it would be pretty likely to destroy the fecundating property of what might remain. But if this check were ever so sure, it would, in my opinion, fall short of being equal, all things considered, to the one I am about to mention— one which not only dislodges the semen pretty effectually, but at the same time destroys the fecundating property of the whole of it.

It consists in syringing the vagina immediately after connec-

*This was a check advocated by Carlile.—[Publishers' note.]

137

tion, with a solution of sulphate of zinc, of alum, pearl-ash, or any salt that acts chemically on the semen, and at the same time produces no unfavorable effect on the female.

In all probability, a vegetable astringent would answer—as an infusion of white oak bark, of red rose leaves, of nut-galls, and the like. A lump of either of the above-mentioned salts, of the size of a chestnut, may be dissolved in a pint of water, making the solution weaker or stronger, as it may be borne without producing any irritation of the parts to which it is applied. These solutions will not lose their virtues by age. A female syringe, which will be required in the use of the check, may be had at the shop of an apothecary for a shilling or less. If preferred, the semen may be dislodged, as far as it can be, by syringing with simple water, after which some of the solution is to be injected, to destroy the fecundating property of what may remain lodged between the ridges of the vagina, &c.

I know the use of this check requires the woman to leave her bed for a few moments, but this is its only objection; and it would be unreasonable to suppose that any check can ever be devised entirely free of objections. In its favour, it may be said, it costs nearly nothing; it is sure; it requires no sacrifice of pleasure; it is in the hands of the female; it is to be used after, instead of before connection, a weighty consideration in its favour, as a moment's reflection will convince any one; and last, but not least, it is conducive to cleanliness, and preserves the parts from relaxation and disease. The vagina may be very much contracted by a persevering use of astringent injections, and they are constantly used for this purpose in cases of *procidentia uteri*, or a sinking down of the womb—subject as women are to *fluor albus*, and other diseases of the genital organs, it is rather a matter of wonder that they are not more so, considering the prevailing practices. Those who have used this check (and some have used it, to my certain knowledge, with entire success for nine or ten years, and under such circumstances as leave no room to doubt its efficacy) affirm they would be at the trouble of using injections merely for the purposes of health and cleanliness.*

*There is no doubt that many diseases of the female organs might be

By actual experiment it has been rendered highly probable that pregnancy may, in many instances, be prevented by injections of simple water, applied with a tolerable degree of care. But simple water has failed, and its occasional failure is what we should expect, considering the anatomy of the parts, and the results of Spallanzani's experiments heretofore alluded to.

Thus much did I say respecting this check in the first edition of this work. That is what I call the chemical check. The idea of destroying the fecundating property of the semen was original, if it did not originate with me. My attention was drawn to the subject by the perusal of "Moral Physiology." Such was my confidence in the chemical idea, that I sat down and wrote this work in July, 1831. But the reflection that I did not know that this check would never fail, and that if it should I might do some one an injury in recommending it, caused the manuscript to lie on hand until the following December. Some time in November I fell in with an old acquaintance, who agreeably surprised me by stating that to his own personal knowledge this last check had been used as above stated. I have since conversed with a gentleman with whom I was acquainted, who stated that, being in Baltimore some few years ago, he was there informed of this check by those who have no doubt of its efficacy. From what has as yet fell under my own observation, I am not warranted in drawing any conclusion. I can only say I have not known it to fail. Such are my views on the whole subject, that it would require many instances of its reputed failure to satisfy me that such failures were not owing to an insufficient use of it. I even believe that quite cold water alone, if thoroughly used, would be sufficient. In Spallanzani's experiments warm water was unquestionably used. As the seminal animalculae are essential to impregnation, all we have to do is to change the condition of, or, if you will, to kill them; and, as they are so exceedingly small and delicate, this is doubtless easily done, and hence cold water may be sufficient.

What has now been advanced in this work will enable the reader to judge for himself or herself of the efficacy of the chem-

prevented by greater personal cleanliness, and by the use of the syringe.—[Publishers' note.]

ical or syringe check, and time will probably determine whether I am correct in this matter. I do know that those married females who have much desire to escape will not stand for the little trouble of using this check, especially when they consider that on the score of cleanliness and health alone, it is worth all this trouble.

A great part of the time no check is necessary, and women of experience and observation with the information conveyed by this work will be able to judge pretty correctly when it is and when it is not. They may rest assured that none of the salts mentioned will have any deleterious effect. The sulphate of zinc is commonly known by the name of white vitriol. This, as well as alum, have been extensively used for leucorrhoea. Acetate of lead would doubtless be effectual—indeed, it has proved to be so; but I do not recommend it, because I conceive it possible that a long-continued use of it might impair the instinct.

I hope that no failures will be charged to inefficacy of this check which ought to be attributed to negligence or insufficient use of it. I will therefore recommend at least two applications of the syringe, the sooner the surer, yet it is my opinion that five minutes' delay would not prove michievous—perhaps not ten.

CHAPTER IV

## Remarks on the Reproductive Instinct

I SCARCELY need observe that by this instinct is meant the desire for sexual intercourse. Blumenbach speaks of this instinct as "superior to all others in universality and violence." Perhaps hunger is an exception. But surely no instinct commands a greater proportion of our thoughts, or has a greater influence upon our happiness for better or for worse. "Controlled by reason and chastened by good feeling, it gives to social intercourse much of its charm and zest, but directed by selfishness or governed by force it is prolific of misery and degradation. In itself, it appears to be the most social and least selfish of all instincts. It fits us to give even while receiving pleasure, and among cultivated beings the former power is even more highly valued than the latter. Not one of our instincts perhaps affords larger scope for the exercise of disinterestedness or fitter play for the best moral feelings of our race. Not one gives birth to relations more gentle, more humanising and endearing, not one lies more immediately at the root of the kindliest charities and most generous impulses that honour and bless human nature. It is a much more noble, because less purely selfish, instinct than hunger or thirst. It is an instinct that entwines itself around the warmest feelings and best affections of the heart."—*Moral Physiology*. But too frequently its strength, together with a want of moral culture, is such that it is not "controlled by reason;" and consequently, from time immemorial, it has been gratified, either in a michievous manner, or to such an intemperate degree, or under such improper circumstances, as to give rise to an incalculable amount of human misery. For this reason it has, by some, been regarded as a low, degrading, and "carnal" passion, with which a holy life must be ever at war. But, in the instinct itself, the philosopher sees nothing deserving of degrading epithets. He sees not that nature should war against herself. He believes that in savage life it *is*, and in wisely organized societies of duly enlightened and civilized beings it *would be*, a source of tenfold more happiness than misery.

A part of the evil consequences to which this instinct is daily giving rise under the present state of things, it belongs more particularly to the moralist to point out; whilst of others it falls within the province of the physician to treat. But let me first remark, that physicians have hitherto fallen far short of giving those instructions concerning this instinct which its importance demands. In books, pamphlets, journals, &c., they have laid much before the public respecting eating, drinking, bathing, lacing, air, exercise, &c.; but have passed by the still more important subject now before us, giving only here and there some faint allusion to it. This, it is true, the customs, not to say pruderies, of the age, have compelled them to do, in publications designed for the public eye, yet, in some small work, indicated by its title to be for private perusal, they might, with the utmost propriety,

have embodied much highly useful instruction in relation to this
instinct.*

This instinct is liable to be gratified at improper times, to an
intemperate degree, and in a mischievous manner.

True philosophy dictates that this and all other appetites be so
gratified as will most conduce to human happiness—not merely
the happiness attending the gratification of one of the senses, but
all the senses—not merely sensual happiness, but intellectual—
not merely the happiness of the individual, but of the human
family.

First.—Of the times at which this instinct ought not to be
gratified. With females it ought not to be gratified until they are
seventeen or eighteen years of age, and with males not until they
are a year or two older. The reason is, if they refrain until these
ages, the passion will hold out the longer, and they will be able to
derive much more pleasure from it in after life, than if earlier
gratified, especially to any great extent. A due regard to health
also enjoins with most persons some restraint on this instinct—
indeed, at all times, but especially for a few years after the
above-mentioned ages. It ought not to be rashly gratified at first.
Begin temperately, and as the system becomes more mature, and
more habituated to the effects naturally produced by the gratification of this instinct, it will bear more without injury. Many
young married people, ignorant of the consequences, have debilitated the whole system—the genital system in particular; have
impaired their mental energies; have induced consumptive and
other diseases; have rendered themselves irritable, unsocial, melancholy, and finally, much impaired, perhaps destroyed their affection for each other, by an undue gratification of the
reproductive instinct. In almost all diseases, if gratified at all, it
should be very temperately. It ought not to be gratified during
menstruation, as it might prove productive, to the man, of symptoms similar to those of syphilis,† but more probably to the

*Since this was written many such popular medical works have been is-
sued and publicly sold.—[Publishers' note.]

†Gonorrhoea, or a purulent discharge, and not syphilis, is evidently what
is here meant by Dr. Knowlton. The two affections were at one time confounded together, and were often thought to be different forms of the same
disease, but they are now known to be quite distinct. Syphilis is the product

woman of a weakening disease called *fluor albus*. In case of pregnancy a temperate gratification for the first two or three months may be of no injury to the woman or the forthcoming offspring. But it ought to be known that the growth of the foetus in utero may be impaired, and the seeds of future bodily infirmity and mental imbecility of the offspring may be sown, by much indulgence during utero-gestation or pregnancy, especially when the woman experiences much pleasure in such indulgences.

Having already glanced at some of the bad effects of an undue gratification of this instinct, I have but little more to offer under the head of Intemperate Degree. It will be borne in mind that temperance in this thing is not to be decided by numbers, but that it depends on circumstances; and what would be temperance in one, may be intemperance in another. And with respect to an individual, too, what he might enjoy with impunity, were he a labouring man, or a man whose business requires but little mental exercise, would, were he a student, unfit him for the successful prosecution of his studies. Intemperance in the gratification of this instinct has a tendency to lead to intemperance in the use of ardent spirits. The langour, depression of spirits, in some instances faintness and want of appetite, induced by intemperate gratification, call loudly for some stimulus, and give a relish to spirits. Thus the individual is led to drink. This inflames the blood, the passions, and leads to further indulgence. This again calls for more spirits; and thus two vicious habits are commenced, which mutually increase each other. Strange as it may appear to those unacquainted with the animal economy, an intemperate indulgence sometimes gives rise to the same disease— so far as the name makes it so—that is frequently cured by a temperate indulgence; viz., nocturnal emissions.

Every young married woman ought to know that the male system is exhausted in a far greater degree than the female by gratification. It seems, indeed, to have but little effect, comparatively, upon some females. But with respect to the male, it has been estimated by Tissot that the loss of one ounce of semen

---

of a peculiar blood-poison, and never arises except by contagion from another person suffering from a similar disease.—G. R.

is equal in its effects upon the system to the loss of 40 ounces of blood. As it respects the immediate effects, this estimation, generally speaking may not be too great. But a man living on a full meat diet might, doubtless, part with fifty ounces of semen in the course of a year, with far less detriment to the system than with 2000 ounces of blood. It is a fact, that mode of living independent of occupation makes a great difference with respect to what the system will bear. A full meat diet, turtles, oysters, eggs, spirits, wine, &c., certainly promote the secretion of semen, and enable the system to bear its emission. But a cool vegetable and milk diet calms all the fiercer passions, the venereal especially. Most men adopting such a diet as this will suffer no inconvenience in extending the intervals of their gratification to three or four weeks; on the contrary, they will enjoy clear intellect, and a fine flow of spirits. This is the diet for men of literary pursuits, especially the unmarried.

As to the mischievous manner, it consists in the unnatural habit of onanism, or solitary gratification; it is an anti-social and demoralising habit, which, while it proves no quietus to the mind, impairs the bodily powers, as well as mental, and not unfrequently leads to insanity.

While the gratification of the reproductive instinct in such manner as I have mentioned leads to bad consequences, a temperate and natural gratification, under proper circumstances, is attended with good—besides the mere attendant pleasure, which alone is enough to recommend such gratification. I admit that human beings might be so constituted that if they had no reproductive instinct to gratify, they might enjoy good health; but being constituted as they are, this instinct cannot be mortified with impunity. It is a fact universally admitted, that unmarried females do not enjoy so much good health and attain to so great an age as the married; notwithstanding that the latter are subject to the diseases and pains incident to child-bearing. A temperate gratification promotes the secretions, and the appetite for food; calms the restless passions; induces pleasant sleep; awakens social feeling, and adds a zest to life which makes one conscious that life is worth preserving.

## APPENDIX

[I here connect with this work, by way of Appendix, the following extract from an article which appeared in the "Boston Investigator," a paper which, *mirabile dictu,* is so "crazy" as to be open to the investigation of all subjects which mightily concern mankind.]

THE only seeming objection of much weight that can be brought against diffusing a knowledge of checks is, that it will serve to increase illegal connections. Now this is exactly the contrary effect of that which those who have diffused such knowledge most confidently believe will arise from it. To diminish such connection is indeed one of the grand objects of these publications—an object which laws and prisons cannot, or at least do not, accomplish. Why is there so much prostitution in the land? The true answer to the question is not, and never will be—Because the people have become acquainted with certain facts in physiology. It is because there are so many unmarried men and women—men of dissipation and profligacy, owing to their not having married in their younger days and settled down in life. But why are there so many unmarried people in the country? Not because young hearts, when they arrive at the age of maturity, do not desire to marry, but because prudential considerations interfere. The young man thinks I cannot marry yet, I cannot support a family, I must make money first, and think of a matrimonial settlement afterwards. And so it is that, through fear of having a family, before they have made a little head-way in the world, and of being thereby compelled to "tug at the oar of incessant labour throughout their lives," thousands of young men do not marry, but go abroad into the world, and form vicious acquaintances and practices. The truth, then, is this, there is so much of illegal connection in the land, because the people had not, twenty years ago, that very information which, it would seem, to some, doubtless through want of due reflection, are apprehensive will increase this evil. I might quote pages to the point from "Every Woman's Book;" but I fear my communication would be too lengthy. I content myself with a few lines. "But when it has become the custom here as elsewhere to limit the number of children, so that none need have more than they wish, no man will fear to take a wife, all will marry while young; debauchery will diminish; while good morals, and religious duties will be promoted."

It has been asked, if a general knowledge of checks would not diminish the general increase of population? I think that such would not be the result in this country until such result would be desirable. In my opinion, the effect would be a good many more families (and on the whole as many births), but not so many overgrown and poverty-stricken ones.

It has been said, it is best to let nature take her course. Now in the broadest sense of the word nature, I say so too. In this sense, there is nothing unnatural in the universe. But if we limit the sense of the word nature so as not to include what we mean by art, then is civilized life one continued warfare against nature. It is by art that we subdue the forest, by art we contend against the elements; by art we combat the natural tendency of disease, &c.

As to the outrageous slander which here and there one has been heard to utter against the fair sex, in saying that fear of conception is the foundation of their chastity, it must be the sentiment of a "carnal heart," which has been peculiarly unfortunate in its acquaintances. 'To the pure all things are pure.' Chastity, as well as its opposite, is in a great degree constitutional; and ought in a like degree to be regarded as a physical property, if I may so say, rather than a moral quality. Where the constitution is favourable, a very indifferent degree of moral training is sufficient to secure the virgin without the influence of the above-mentioned fear; but where it is the reverse, you may coop up the individual in the narrow dark cage of ignorance and fear, as you will, but still you must watch. An eminent moralist has said, "That chastity which will not bear the light [of Physiology] is scarcely worth preserving." But, verily, I believe there is very little such in the market. What there be is naturally short-lived, and, after its demise, the unhappily constituted individual stands in great need of this light to save her from ignominy. What might it not have prevented in the Fall River affair? And if one of two things must happen, either the destruction of fecundity or the destruction of life, which of the two is the greater evil? In these cases, alone, this light is calculated to do sufficient good to counterbalance all the evil that would arise from it; so that we should have its important advantages to the married, in a political, a domestic, and a medical point of view, as so much clear gain. This of course is my opinion; but since I have probably reflected more upon the subject than all the persons concerned in my imprisonment put together, until it can be shown that I have not as clear a head and as pure a heart as any of them, I think it entitled to some weight.

FINIS.

THE

# LAW OF POPULATION:

## ITS CONSEQUENCES,

### AND

### Its Bearing upon Human Conduct and Morals.

BY

## ANNIE BESANT.

[NINETIETH THOUSAND.]

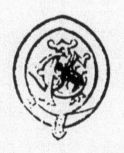

LONDON:

FREETHOUGHT PUBLISHING COMPANY,

63, FLEET STREET, E.C.

1884.

PRICE SIXPENCE

## PREFACE TO SEVENTIETH THOUSAND
## ENGLISH EDITION, 1882

FOUR-AND-A-HALF years have passed away since this little book was first issued; it was written for the poor, in the hope that by the information therein given—information long familiar to and long acted upon by the wealthier classes of society—poor men and women might make the home happy, and rear in respectability and comfort a limited number of children, children who should hereafter bless the parents whose wisdom and forethought had given them a fair chance in the life-race. That hope has been largely realised. During these years fifty thousand copies of the book have found their way into English homes; across the Atlantic it has found warm welcome, and very large American editions have been sold. It has been translated into German, Italian, French, Swedish, and Dutch, and has thus spread over the Continent of Europe, while the English edition has been largely sold in Hindustan, Australia, and New Zealand. A circulation so wide is the sign of the need which this pamphlet has striven to supply. Everywhere men and women are struggling for life; everywhere the labor market is overcrowded and the workers are starving; no longer are the masses content to labor and die without effort to change their condition; education is spreading, and men in becoming rational become prudent and far-seeing. Parents see the labor market over-crowded to-day, and can calculate the result of large families growing up in the near future, so that ten shall fight for the work which is already too little for two. Hence the determination to limit the number of the family within the means of sustaining it in decency and in comfort.

This growing determination has been largely spread by the work of the Malthusian League. This body was founded to defend and promulgate the doctrine of early marriage, parental responsibility, and limitation of the family. By tracts, leaflets, and lectures these doctrines have been taught from one end of the United Kingdom to the other; doctors and clergymen are found within the ranks of these workers for humanity; wives and mothers have pressed in to aid in the good work. To the President of the League, C. Drysdale, M.D., the poor owe large debt of thanks, and in the days to come his name will not be unremembered by those to whom he has devoted his means and his life.

The progress made by the views advocated in this pamphlet has been startingly rapid. At first no words were too strong to hurl against the audacious teachers of doctrines offensive to the wealthy although welcomed by the poor. Mr. Truelove was imprisoned for selling a publication identical in object with the present work, and Sir George Jessel, the Master of the Rolls, thought no words too coarse and too brutal for condemnation of myself. Today, all thoughtful people are recognising the absolute necessity of grappling with the growing poverty of the masses, and the leading journals even of London, deprecate the reckless multiplication which renders nugatory all attempts to cure the sore of pauperism. People are beginning to understand that some change must be made; they see France growing in prosperity, peaceful and contented, and they see the threatening socialism of Germany; they contrast the conjugal prudence of the French with the conjugal recklessness of the German; they note the birth-rate of the two countries, and see therein one of the reasons for the contrast. They see the high birth-rate of England and of Ireland, the constant strain of living, the scarcity of work and of food. Rational human beings cannot fold their arms idly in face of these perils, and they are gradually accepting as an axiom the doctrines which they at first repelled with scorn.

"The world moves," and it moves onward. Early marriage and limitation of the family mean growth of social purity and of home happiness among the people. The bigots and the persecutors may, if they will, still fight against the inevitable, but the people have caught a glimpse of the path, out of poverty and none can turn them back. Persecution has only popularised our doctrines. The first issue of this little book was a rallying flag held firmly in the whirl of the struggle; the present issue of the seventieth thousand is the triumphal flag planted on the citadel which has been won from the foe.

ANNIE BESANT

In issuing another twenty thousand of this little book, I have nothing to add to the above.—A. B., 1884.

## The Law of Population

THE law of population first laid down in this country by the Rev. T. R. Malthus in his great work entitled "The Principle of Population," has long been known to every student, and accepted by every thinker. It is, however, but very recently that this question has become ventilated among the many, instead of being discussed only by the few. Acknowledged as an axiom by the naturalist and by the political economist, the law of population has never been appreciated by the mass of the people. The free press pioneers of the last generation, Richard Carlile, James Watson, Robert Dale Owen—these men had seen its importance and had endeavored, by cheap publications dealing with it from its practical side, to arouse attention and to instruct those for whom they worked. But the lesson fell on stony ground and passed almost unheeded; it would, perhaps, be fairer to say that the fierce political conflicts of the time threw all other questions into a comparative shade; nor must the strong prejudice against Malthus be forgotten—the prejudice which regarded him as a hard, cold theorist, who wrote in the interest of the richer classes, and would deny to the poor man the comfort of wife and home. The books issued at this period—such as Carlile's "Every Woman's Book," Knowlton's "Fruits of Philosophy," R. D. Owen's "Moral Physiology"—passed unchallenged by authority, but obtained only a limited circulation; here and there they did their work, and the result was seen in the greater comfort and respectability of the families who took advantage of their teachings; but the great mass of the people went on in their ignorance and their ever-increasing poverty, conscious that mouths multiply more rapidly than wages, but dimly supposing that Providence was the responsible agent, and that where "God sends mouths" he ought to "send meat." One or two recognised advocates for the people did not forget the social side of the work which they had inherited; men like Austin Holyoake and Charles Bradlaugh, carrying on the struggle of Carlile and Watson, were not careless of this vital portion of it, and Mr. Holyoake's "Large and Small Families," and Mr. Bradlaugh's declaration that the *National Reformer* was to be "Malthusian" in its political economy, proved that these two, at least, were sound on this scarcely regarded branch of social science.

Now, all has changed; Malthusianism has become one of the "burning questions" of the day, and a low-priced work, stating clearly the outlines of the subject, has become a necessity. Our paternal authorities, like their predecessors, entertain a horror of cheap knowledge, but they will have to assent to the circulation of cheap information on social science, as those who went before them were compelled to tacitly assent to cheap information touching kings and priests.

The law of population, tersely stated, is—"there is a tendency in all animated existence to increase faster than the means of subsistence." Nature produces more life than she can support, and the superabundant life is kept down by the want of food. Malthus put the law thus: "The constant tendency in all animated life to increase beyond the nourishment prepared for it." "It is observed by Dr. Franklin," he writes, "that there is no bound to the prolific nature of plants or animals but what is made by their crowding and interfering with each other's means of subsistence. . . . . Throughout the animal and vegetable kingdoms, nature has scattered the seeds of life abroad with the most profuse and liberal hand; but has been comparatively sparing in the room and the nourishment necessary to rear them." "Population," Malthus teaches, "when unchecked, goes on doubling itself every twenty-five years;" "in the northern States of America, where the means of subsistence have been more ample, the manners of the people more pure, and the checks to early marriages fewer than in any of the modern States of Europe, the population has been found to double itself, for above a century and a half successively, in less than twenty-five years. . . . . In the back settlements, where the sole employment is agriculture, and vicious customs and unwholesome occupations are little known, the population has been found to double itself in fifteen years. Even this extraordinary rate of increase is probably short of the utmost power of population."

The "power of increase" of the human species, according to John Stuart Mill, "is indefinite, and the actual multiplication would be extraordinarily rapid, if the power were exercised to the utmost. It never is exercised to the utmost, and yet, in the most favorable circumstances known to exist, which are those of a fertile region colonised from an industrious and civilised community, population has continued for several generations, independently of fresh immigration, to double itself in not much more than twenty years . . . . It is a very low estimate of the capacity of increase, if we only assume that in a good sanitary condition of the people, each generation may be double the number of the generation which preceded it." James Mill wrote: "That population therefore has such a tendency to increase as would enable it to double itself in a small number of years, is a proposition resting on the strongest evidence, which nothing that deserves the name of evidence has been brought on the other side to oppose."

Mr. McCulloch tells us that "it has been established beyond all question that the population of some of the states of North America, after making due allowance for immigration, has continued to double for a century past in so short a period as twenty, or at most five-and-twenty, years." M. Moreau De Jonnès gives us the following table of the time in which the population of each of the under-mentioned countries would double itself:—

| Turkey | would take | ... | ... | 555 years |
|---|---|---|---|---|
| Switzerland | " | ... | ... | 227 " |
| France | " | ... | ... | 138 " |
| Spain | " | ... | ... | 106 " |
| Holland | " | ... | ... | 100 " |

| Germany | would take | ... | ... | 76 years |
|---|---|---|---|---|
| Russia | " | ... | ... | 43 " |
| England | " | ... | ... | 43 " |
| United States | " | ... | ... | 25 " |

(Without reckoning immigrants.)

We shall take but a narrow view of the law of population if we confine ourselves exclusively to human beings. Man is but the highest in the animal kingdom, not a creature apart from it, and the law of population runs through the animal and vegetable worlds. To take the commonest illustration: the horse is but a slowly breeding animal, producing but one at a birth, and that at considerable intervals of time; yet how small a proportion of the horses of a country are either stallions or brood mares; the reproductive organs of the colt are destroyed in the enormous majority of those born, and, nevertheless, our production of horses suffices for the vast needs of our commercial and luxurious classes. Darwin, in his "Origin of Species," writes:—"There is no exception to the rule that every organic being naturally increases at so high a rate that, if not destroyed, the earth would soon be covered by the progeny of a single pair. Even slow-breeding man has doubled in twenty-five years, and at this rate, in a few thousand years, there would literally not be room for his progeny. Linnaeus has calculated that if an annual plant produced only two seeds—and there is no plant so unproductive as this—and their seedlings next year produced two and so on, then in twenty years there would be a million plants. The elephant is reckoned the slowest breeder of all known animals, and I have taken some pains to estimate its probable minimum rate of natural increase; it will be under the mark to assume that it breeds when thirty years old, and goes on breeding till ninety years old, bringing forth three pair of young in this interval; if this be so, at the end of the fifth century there would be alive 15,000,000 elephants, descended from the first pair. But we have better evidence on this subject than mere theoretical calculations, namely, the numerous recorded cases of the astonishingly rapid increase of various animals in a state of nature, when circumstances have been favorable to them during two or three following seasons. Still more striking is the evidence from our domestic animals of many kinds which have run wild in many parts of the world; if the statements of the rate of increase of slow-breeding cattle and horses in South America, and latterly in Australia, had not been well authenticated, they would have been incredible. So it is with plants; cases could be given of introduced plants which have become common throughout whole islands in a period of less than ten years. Several of the plants, such as the cardoon and a tall thistle, now most numerous over the wide plains of La Plata, clothing square leagues of surface almost to the exclusion of all other plants, have been introduced from Europe; and there are plants which now range in India, as I hear from Dr. Falconer, from Cape Comorin to the Himalayas, which have been imported from America since its discovery. In such cases, and endless instances could be given, no one supposes that the fertility of these animals or plants has been suddenly and temporarily increased in any sensible degree. The obvious explanation is that the conditions of life have been very favorable, and that there has consequently been less destruction of the old and young, and that nearly all the young have been enabled to breed. In such cases the geometrical ratio of increase, the result of which never fails to be surprising, simply explains the extraordinary rapid increase and wide diffusion of naturalised productions in their new homes. In a state of nature almost every plant produces seed, and amongst animals there are very few which do not annually pair. Hence, we may confidently assert that all plants and animals are tending to increase at a geometrical ratio, that all would most rapidly stock every station in which they could anyhow exist, and that the geometrical tendency to increase must be checked by destruction at some period of life."

Mr. John Stuart Mill also remarks: "The power of multiplication inherent in all organic life may be regarded as *infinite*. There is no species of vegetable or animal, which, if the earth were entirely abandoned to it, and to the things on which it feeds, would not in a small number of years overspread every region of the globe of which the climate was compatible with its existence."

The rapid multiplication of rabbits in Australia has lately given a startling instance of reproductive power; a number of rabbits were taken over and let loose; the district was thinly peopled, so they were not shot down to any great extent; their natural enemies, the hawks, weasels, etc., that prey on their young in England, were not taken over with them; food was abundant, and there was no check to keep them back; the consequence was that whole districts were overrun by them, and the farmers were at their wits' end to save their crops from the swarming rodents. In France, again, owing to the wholesale destruction of small birds, there was a perfect plague of insects, and the inhabitants of many districts have striven to import birds, so as to prevent the insects from practically destroying the vegetation.

While in the vegetable and animal kingdoms the rapidity of the increase is generally far greater than in the human race, we have yet seen how rapidly man has been found to increase where the circumstances surrounding him were favorable to vigorous life. We have never yet, however, seen the full power of reproduction among mankind; the increase of population in America "falls very far short," says the author of the "Elements of Social Science," "of the possible rate of increase, as is seen by the short average of life in America, and by the large amount of the reproductive power which, even in that country, is lost from celibacy and prostitution. . . . . The capacity of increase in the human race, as in all other organised beings, is, in fact, boundless and immeasurable."

But while animated existence increases thus rapidly, no such swift multiplication can be secured of the means of subsistence. The means of subsistence of vegetable life are strictly limited in quantity; the amount obtainable from the soil may be increased by manure, by careful tillage, by rotation of crops, by improved methods of husbandry, but none the less is this amount limitable, while there is no limit to the power of life-production; if the soil and air and light could be indefinitely stretched, vegetable life would still suffice without effort to clothe the increased surface. But since the size of the globe inexorably limits the amount of vegetable produce possible of growth, the limited vegetable produce must, in its turn, limit the amount of animal life which can be sustained. While increased knowledge, skill and care may augment the means of subsistence obtainable from the earth, yet animal life multiplies more rapidly than can its food. As is truly said by the author just quoted: "From a consideration of the law of agricultural industry, and an estimate of the rate at which the means of subsistence could be increased in old countries, even under the most favorable circumstances, it may be inferred with certainty that these means of subsistence could not possibly be increased so fast as to permit population to increase at its natural rate. . . . Let us apply the American rate of increase to the population of this country. Is it conceivably possible that the population of England or any old country should double itself every twenty-five years? In Great Britain there are now" (the book was written many years ago) "about twenty-one millions; is it conceivable that the means of subsistence could be so rapidly increased as to allow these twenty-one millions to swell to forty-two millions in the first twenty-five years; to eighty-four millions in the next; 168 millions in the next, &c.? The supposition is evidently absurd. Even the rate of increase of the last fifty-three years (in which time the population has doubled) cannot possibly be long continued. If it were, it would increase our population in three centuries to about 1,300 millions; or, in other words, to more than the total population of the globe, which is estimated at about 1,000 millions."

Wherever, then, we look throughout Nature, we find proofs of the truth of the law, that "there is a tendency in all animated existence to increase faster than the means of subsistence." This is the law of which Miss Martineau said that it could be no more upset than a law of arithmetic; this is the law which John Stuart Mill regarded "as axiomatic;" this is the law which the Lord Chief Justice designated "an irrefragable truth." Controversialists may quarrel as to its consequences, and may differ as to man's duty in regard to them, but no controversy can arise among thinkers on the law itself, any more than on the sphericity of the earth.

CHAPTER II

## Its Consequences

IT IS abundantly clear, from experience, that population does not, as a general rule, increase at anything like the rate spoken of in the preceding chapter. The earth would, long ere now, have become unable to support her offspring if they had multiplied at the pace which the naturalist tells us is possible—if, for instance, all rabbits had increased in the same ratio as those taken over to Australia and naturalised there. Some cause must therefore be at work checking the increase and preventing over-rapid multiplication, holding the balance, in fact, roughly even between the means of subsistence and the living creatures who consume them. In the vegetable kingdom the checks to increase are not difficult to find. Every plant needs for its development suitable soil, moisture, air, and light; these are its means of subsistence. The amount of these is limited, while the power of multiplication in the vegetable is unlimited. What is the necessary consequence? That of the myriad seeds produced only a few will develop into seed-bearing plants; each seed needs a certain proportion of soil, moisture, air, light; if they fall round the parent stem and sprout into seedlings they so crowd each other that the weaker perish; every gardener knows that his seedlings need thinning if any are to grow into useful plants, that his plantations must be thinned out if any tree is to have full development; an over-crowded plantation, an over-crowded garden-bed, gives a crop of dwarfed, stunted, weak, and useless plants. These facts are so commonplace that they pass continually before our eyes, and the simple inference from them is unregarded. There is another check of a severe character on vegetable increase. Birds eat the seeds; animals browse on the plants; man uses many kinds for his own support; the wheat sown in one year not only produces the seed-corn for the ensuing season, but also affords so vast a multiplication as to supply the world with bread; the animal world preys on the vegetable, and so is made a check which destroys the mature, as well as the check of want of room and nourishment which destroys the infant, growth. Out of 357 seedlings of English weeds, carefully watched by Mr. Darwin, 295 were destroyed. On some heaths near Farnham, in the portions enclosed during ten years previously, self-sown firs were observed by him springing up so closely that all could not live, while in the unenclosed portions not one young tree was to be seen. On close examination Mr. Darwin found in one square yard thirty-two little trees no higher than the heather, one with twenty-six rings of growth; the check here was the browsing of cattle over the open part of the heath. In the animal kingdom the same class of checks is found; the rabbit which in Australia has become an intolerable plague, is kept down to a fair level in England, not because he multiplies less rapidly, but because the check of destruction is brought to bear upon him; food is scarcer in the more cultivated land; guns and traps send him to the market in millions; hawks, weasels, cats, prey upon his young; he produces life rapidly, but the check of death waits upon him and keeps him down. The swift increase of plants and animals under favorable circumstances, dealt with in Chapter I, shows the enormous power of the destructive checks which generally keep in subjection the life-producing force. Once more turning to Mr. Darwin, we read:—

"Of the many individuals of any species which are periodically born, but a small number can survive.... A struggle for existence inevitably follows from the high rate at which all organic beings tend to increase. Every being, which during its natural lifetime produces several eggs or seeds, must suffer destruction during some period of its life, and during some season or occasional year, otherwise on the principle of geometrical increase, its numbers would quickly become so inordinately great that no country could support the product. Hence, as more individuals are produced than can possibly survive, there must in every case be a struggle for existence, either one individual with another of the same species, or with the individuals of distinct species, or with the physical conditions of life. It is the doctrine of Malthus applied with manifold force to the whole animal and vegetable kingdoms; for in this case there can be no artificial increase of food, and no prudential restraint from marriage. Although some species may be now increasing more or less rapidly in numbers, all cannot do so, for the world would not hold them. ... Our familiarity with the larger domestic animals tends, I think, to mislead us; we see no great destruction falling on them, and we forget that thousands are annually slaughtered for food, and that in a state of nature an equal number would have somehow to be disposed of. ... In looking at nature, it is most necessary to keep the foregoing considerations always in mind—never to forget that every single organic being around us may be said to be striving to the utmost to increase in numbers; that each lives by a struggle at some period of its life; that heavy destruction inevitably falls either on the young or old during each generation or at recurrent intervals. Lighten any check, mitigate the destruction ever so little, and the number of the species will almost instantaneously increase to any amount."

If there be such vast destruction of life throughout the vegetable and animal kingdoms, necessarily consequent on the superabundance of life produced, is man exempt from the same law?

Malthus laid down the three following propositions, propositions of which this book is only an amplification:—

"1. Population is necessarily limited by the means of subsistence.

"2. Population invariably increases where the means of subsistence increase, unless prevented by some very powerful and obvious checks.

"3. These checks, and the checks which repress the superior power of population, and keep its effects on a level with the means of subsistence, are all resolvable into moral restraint, vice, and misery.

"The ultimate check to population appears to be a want of food, arising necessarily from the different ratios according to which population and food increase. But this ultimate check is never the immediate check, except in cases of actual famine. The immediate check may be stated to consist in all those customs and all those diseases, which seem to be generated by a scarcity of the means of subsistence; and all those causes, independent of this scarcity, whether of a moral or physical nature, which tend prematurely to weaken and destroy the human frame." These causes which retard the growth of population by killing human beings, either slowly or rapidly, are all classed together by Malthus under the head of "positive" checks; they are the "natural" checks to population, common alike to vegetables, to animals, to man; they are all checks of suffering, of want, of disease; they are life-destroying, anti-human, brutal, irrational.

These checks are, as might be imagined, more striking, more openly repulsive, more thorough, among savage than among civilised nations. War, infanticide, hardship, famine, disease, murder of the aged, all these are among the positive checks which keep down the increase of population among savage tribes. War carries off the young men, full of vigor, the warriors in their prime of life, the strongest, the most robust, the most fiery— those, in fact, who, from their physical strength and energy would be most likely to add largely to the number of the tribe. Infanticide, most prevalent where means of existence are most restricted, is largely practised among barbarous nations, the custom being due, to a great extent, to the difficulty of providing food for a large family. Hardship carries away many a child in savage life: "Women," says Malthus, "obliged, by their habits of living, to a constant change of places, and compelled to unremitting drudgery for their husbands, appear to be absolutely incapable of bringing up two or three children nearly of the same age. If another child be born before the one above it can shift for itself, and follow its mother on foot, one of the two must almost necessarily perish from want of care." Famine, so easily caused among a primitive community, sweeps off young and old together; epidemics carry away almost a whole tribe at one swoop; the aged are often slain, or left to perish, when their feebleness no longer permits them to add to the productive force of the community.

All these miseries are the positive and natural checks to population among uncivilised beings; among the more civilised the checks are the same in kind although more decently veiled. But the moment we come among civilised nations a new factor is introduced into the problem which complicates it very considerably. Hitherto we have seen Nature—apart from man—going her own way, producing and destroying without let or hindrance. But when we examine civilised nations we find a new agent at work; Nature's grandest product, the brain of man, now comes into play, and a new set of circumstances arises. Men, women, and children, who would be doomed to death in the savage state, have their lives prolonged by civilisation; the sickly, whom the hardships of the savage struggle for existence would kill off, are carefully tended in hospitals, and saved by medical skill; the parents, whose thread of life would be cut short, are cherished on into prolonged old age; the feeble, who would be left to starve, are tenderly shielded from hardship, and life's road is made the smoother for the lame; the average of life is lengthened, and more and more thought is brought to bear on the causes of preventible disease; better drainage, better homes, better food, better clothing, all these, among the more comfortable classes, remove many of the natural checks to population. Among these nations wars become less frequent and less bloody; famines, owing to improved means of intercommunication, become for a time almost impossible; epidemics no longer depopulate whole districts. In England, in A.D. 1258, no less than 15,000 people were starved to death in London alone; in France, in A.D. 1348, one-third of the whole population perished from the same cause; in Rome, from A.D. 250–265, a plague raged, that, for some time, carried off daily 5,000 persons; in England, in A.D. 1506 and 1517, the sweating sickness slew half the inhabitants of the large towns and depopulated Oxford; in London, in A.D. 1603–4, the plague killed 30,578 persons, and in A.D. 1664–5 it destroyed 68,596; in Naples, in A.D. 1656, 400,000 died, and in Egypt, A.D. 1792, above 800,000. These terrible epidemics and famines have ceased to sweep over Europe, but for how long? This decrease of natural checks to population, consequent on advancing civilisation, has, unfortunately, a very dark side. Darwin has remarked: "Lighten any check, mitigate the destruction ever so little, and the number of the species will almost instantaneously increase to any amount." A signal instance of the truth of this remark is now being given to us in our Indian empire by the introduction there of Western civilisation; Lord Derby says: "We have established there order and peace; we have done away with local wars; we have lessened the ravages of pestilence; and we do what we can—and, in ordinary seasons, we do it with success—to mitigate the effects of destitution. The result is, naturally and necessarily, a vast increase in population; and, if present appearances can be trusted, we shall have in every generation a larger aggregate of human beings relying upon us for help in those periods of distress which must, from time to time, occur in a country wholly agricultural and liable to droughts." So that it appears that our civilisation in India, taking away the ordinary natural checks to population, *and introducing no others in their stead,* brings about a famine which has already destroyed more than 500,000 people in one Presidency alone, and has thrown about one and a half million more on charity. From this point of view civilisation can scarcely be regarded as an unmixed blessing, and it must not be forgotten that what is happening in India now must, sooner or later, happen in every country where science destroys the balance of nature.

Turning to England, we find that our population is growing rapidly enough to cause anxiety; although there are some severe checks, with which we shall deal presently, England has almost doubled her population during the last fifty years. In 1810 the population of England and Wales was about 10,000,000, and in 1860 it was about 20,000,000. "At the present time," writes Professor Fawcett, "it is growing at the rate of 200,000 every year, which is almost equivalent to the population of the county of Northampton. If in fifty years the descendants of one million become two millions, it is obvious that in 100 years the two millions will have become four millions, so that if the population of England were eight millions in 1810 it would be 80 millions in 1960." Forty years hence, if we maintain the rate of increase which we have kept up since the commencement of this century, some 40 millions of people will be crowded into our little island; yet "at the present time it is said that there is a great redundancy of labor. Many who are willing to work cannot find employment; in most of our important branches of industry there has been great over-production; every trade and every profession is over-crowded; for every vacant clerkship there are hundreds of applications. Difficult as it is for men to obtain a livelihood, it is ten times more difficult for women to do so; partly on account of unjust laws, and partly because of the tyranny of society, they are shut out from many employments. All that has just been stated is admitted by common consent—it is the topic of daily conversation, and of daily complaint—and yet with the utmost complacency we observe 200,000 added to our population every year, and we often congratulate ourselves upon this addition to our numbers, as if it were an unerring sign of advancing prosperity. But viewed in relation to the facts just mentioned, what does this addition to our numbers indicate? To this question only one reply can be given—that in ten years' time, where there are a hundred now seeking employment there will then be a hundred and twenty. This will not apply simply to one industry, but will be the case throughout the whole country. It will also further happen that in ten years' time for every hundred who now require food, fuel, and clothing, a similar provision will have to be made for one hundred and twenty. It therefore follows that, low as the general average standard of living now is, it cannot by any means be obtained, unless in ten years' time the supply of all the commodities of ordinary consumption can be increased by 20 per cent, without their becoming more costly." The continually rising price of food is one of the most certain signs that population in England is pressing over hard on the means of subsistence; although our own corn and meat production is enormously supplemented by supplies from abroad, prices are always going up, and the large amount of adulteration practised in every food-supplying trade is, to a great extent, an effort to equalise the supply and the demand. Much of the food on which our poor live is unwholesome in the extreme; let anyone walk through the poorer districts of London, or of any large town, and see the provisions lying for sale in the shops; it is not only the meat sold for cooking at home, the doubtful sugar, and not doubtful apology for butter, the blue milk, the limp and flabby vegetables—but let the enquirer stop at the cook-shop and inspect the fish, unpleasant both to eye and smell, in itself and in its cooking; the "faggots"—the eating of which killed a child the other day; the strangely shaped and strangely marked lumps of what should be meat; and, after an hour's walk, the searcher will not wonder at the wan, haggard faces of those who support life on this untempting fare. Even of this fare, however, there is not enough; the low fever so sadly common in poor districts, the "falling away," the hollow cough, the premature old age, all these are the results of insufficiency of food—insufficiency which does not kill at once, but slowly and surely starves away the life. Much of the drunkenness, most common in the poorest districts, has its root in lack of food; the constantly craving stomach is stilled with drink, which it would not desire if it were better filled.

But the pressure on the means of subsistence has other consequences than the living on unwholesome food. One of the earliest signs of too rapidly increasing population is the overcrowding of the poor. Just as the overcrowded seedlings spoil each other's growth, so do the overcrowded poor injure each other morally, mentally, and physically. Whether we study town or country the result of our enquiries is the same—the houses are too small and the families are too large. Take, as illustrating this, the terrible instances given by Mr. George Godwin, in his essay on "Overcrowding in London." In Lincoln Court he states that: "In the majority of the houses the rooms are small, and the staircases are narrow and without ventilation. In two of them it was admitted that more than thirty-five persons lived in each; but it would probably be nearer truth to say that each house of eight rooms contains on an average, including children, forty-five persons." "A child was found dead in Brownlow Street, and on enquiry it was learnt that the mother, a widow, and six children slept in one bed in a small room. The death of the child was attributed to the bedclothes." "In a model lodging house for families, a father, who with his wife and one child occupies one room, has accommodated six of his nine other children the crossway on two camp bedsteads, while three elder girls, one sixteen years old, sleep on a small bedstead near." "In a respectable house not far from the last, occupied by steady artisans and others, I found that nine persons slept in one of the rooms (12 feet by 14 feet), a father, mother and seven children. Eleven shoemakers worked in the attics; and in each of the other five rooms there was a separate family. I could quote scores of such cases of overcrowding in what would seem to be decent houses." "Hundreds of modern houses, built in decent suburban neighborhoods, as if for one family only, are made to contain several. The neat external appearance of many of them gives no suggestion of the dangerously-crowded state of the houses. A description of one of them in Bemerton Street, Caledonian Road, will be more truthful. The basement below the level of the street contains in the front room an old man and his wife; in the back room, two lodgers; in the parlors there are a man and his wife and eight children. On the first floor, a man and his wife and infant; two girls, sixteen and eighteen years of age, and occasionally their mother—all in the front room; and in the small back room, two women, a girl, and two young children. On the second floor, a father, mother, two grown-up sons, an infant, and a brood of rabbits. Two women and two boys in the back room make the whole population of the house thirty-four. In the next there were thirty-three persons similarly divided." "In one small house, with staircase in the centre, there were in the four small rooms on each side of it, forty persons in the daytime. How many there may be at night I cannot say. The atmosphere on the staircase was sickening." Who can wonder that the death-rate is so high in large cities, and that the difference in the death-rate between the rich and poor sections of the same city is appalling? In Glasgow, for the quarter ending June 30th, the death-rate in the Blythswood division was 19; that in the Bridgegate and Wynds division 52½. Many of the deaths in the richer districts might be prevented by better sanitary arrangements and wider sanitary knowledge; the excess in the poorer districts is clearly preventible with our present knowledge, and preventible death is manslaughter. As might be expected, the rate of infant mortality is very high in these overcrowded districts; where 200 children under the age of five years die among the rich, 600 die among the poor; a young child is easily killed, and the bad air and unwholesome food rapidly murder the little ones; again quoting from the Glasgow report: "A large number of the deaths, bearing the relation of 13½ per cent to the total births, were those of children under one year." In addition to the actual deaths caused by over-crowding, we must add to the mass of misery accruing from it, the non-fatal diseases and the general debility and lack of vigorous life so common in our large centres of industry. "Over-crowding," says Mr. Godwin, "means want of pure air; and want of pure air means debility, continued fever, death, widowhood, orphanage, pauperism, and money loss to the living." Epidemics are most fatal in over-crowded districts, not only because they pass so rapidly from one to another, but also because the people dwelling in those districts have less vitality, less vigor of resistance, than those more fortunately circumstanced. "The great reason," said Dr. Drysdale in the late trial in the Court of Queen's Bench, "that typhus fever is so terrible a disease is that people are crowded. It is impossible to have health with large crowded families." Here then is one of the commonest checks to population in all great cities. Nor must the results to morality be omitted in this imperfect summary of the evils which grow out of over-crowding. What modesty, what decency, what self-respect is possible to these men and women, boys and girls, herded together, seven, ten, fourteen in a room? Only the absence of these virtues could make the life endurable for four-and-twenty hours; no delicacy of feeling can exist there, and we cannot wonder at Dr. Drysdale's sad answer in the recent trial: "They do not know what modesty is."

Can there be any doubt that it is the large families so common among the English poor that are at the root of this over-crowding? For not only would the "model-lodging house" spoken of above have been less crowded if the parents, instead of having ten children, had had only two, but with fewer children less money would be needed for food and clothing, and more could be spared for rent. The artisan with six children, forced to live in a stifling pair of rooms in a back street in London in order to be near his work, might, if he had only two, spare money enough to pay his rail to and fro from the suburbs, where the same rent would give him decent accommodation; and not only would he have a better home, but the two children would grow strong in the free air, where the six pine in the London street, and the two would have plenty of food and clothing, where the six lack both. Mr. Godwin recognises this fact; he says: "Amongst the causes which lead to the evil we are deploring we must not overlook the gradual increase of children, while in the case of the laboring man the income mostly remains the same. ... As the children increase in number the wife is prevented from adding by her earnings to the income, and many years must elapse before the children can be put to work." "Ought to be put to work" would be a truer phrase, for the age at which young children are forced to help in winning their daily bread is one of the disgraces of our civilisation.

Overcrowding in country districts is, naturally, not so injurious to health as it is in the towns; the daily work in the open air, the fresh breeze blowing round the cottage, and cleansing, to some extent, the atmosphere within, the fields and lanes where the children can play, all these things may do much to neutralise the harm to health wrought by overcrowding at night. The injury to health caused by large families among the agricultural poor, arises more from other causes than from over-crowding; the low wage cannot pay for a house sufficiently good, and the cheap ill-built cottage, damp, draughty, badly-drained, brings to those who live in it the fever and the ague and the rheumatism so sadly common among these laboring classes. But the moral effect of over-crowding is, as the present Bishop of Manchester said—when serving as the Rev. J. Fraser in the Royal Commission on the employment of children, young persons, and women in agriculture—"fearful to contemplate." "Modesty," he goes on, "must be an unknown virtue, decency an unimaginable thing, where, in one small chamber, with the beds lying as thickly as they can be packed, father, mother, young men, lads, grown and growing up girls—two and sometimes three generations—are herded promiscuously; where every operation of the toilette and of nature—dressings, undressings, births, deaths—is performed by each within the sight or hearing of all; where children of both sexes, to as high an age as twelve or fourteen, or even more, occupy the same bed; where the whole atmosphere is sensual, and human nature is degraded into something below the level of the swine."

The too early putting of the children to work is one of the consequences of over-large families. In the country the children working in gangs in the fields learn evil speech and evil act at an age when they should be innocent, at school and at play. In town, in the factory and in the workroom, the seeds of disease are sown in the child-laborers. "Children in big families," says Dr. Drysdale, "are taken out to work very early, and premature exertion often injures them for life. . . . Children are not fit to do very much work so long as they are half developed, and early death is often the consequence." Children should not work for their bread; the frame is not fit for toil, the brain is not ready for the effort of long attention; those who give the life should support and protect it until the tenderness of childhood is passed away, and the young body is firm-knit and strong, prepared to take its share of the battle, and bear the burden and heat of the day.

From the same pressure and struggle for existence, consequent on the difficulty of winning the means of life in an overcrowded land, arise the unhealthy conditions among which many kinds of work are carried on. Mr. Godwin remarks, as to artificial flower-making: "In an upper room in Oxford Street, not ten feet square, I have seen a dozen delicate young women closely shut up, pursuing this occuption. . . . Many of the workrooms of fashionable milliners are similarly over-crowded, as are those where young girls are engaged in bookstitching. Take, as an example, a house in Fleet Street, looked at not long ago. The

passage is narrow; a door in it shuts with a spring; the staircase
is confined and without ventilation; the atmosphere is steamy
and smells of glue; ascending, it is seen that all the doors shut
with springs. In the first room looked into, forty young women
and girls were sorting and stitching books. . . . Poor creatures so
placed are being slowly slain." Dr. Symes Thompson, writing on
the "Influence of Occupation on Health and Life," points out
the death-bringing circumstances under which too many of our
wealth-producers toil; if there were fewer of them their lives
would be more valuable than they are; horses and cattle are
cared for and protected; the very machinery used is oiled and
polished; only the human machines are worked under life-ruin-
ing conditions, and are left to struggle on as best they may. Dr.
Thompson gives cases of printers—which every one connected
with journalism can supplement by his own experience—where
unwholesome atmosphere and preposterously long hours destroy
the constitution. He tells us how the shoddy-grinders, the cocoa-
matting weavers, the chaff-cutters, the workers in flax, woollen,
and cotton factories, suffer from a "peculiar kind of bronchitis,
arising from the irritation of the dust" and other matters in-
haled, and the cough "is followed by expectoration, and, if the
occupation is continued, emphysema, or, in those predisposed to
phthisis, tubercle is developed." At Sheffield the "inhalation of
metal filings" is "destructive" to the knife and fork grinders, and
although this might be prevented by the use of respirators the
men's lives are not sufficiently valuable to be thus saved. If grit
got into the works of a machine and ruined them the works
would be covered over, but it may pass into men's lungs and kill
them, and no one troubles. Brass-finishers and stone-masons labor under the same disadvantages; lead-poisoning is common
among plumbers, painters, &c.; "women employed in lead works
rarely bear healthy children; in a large number of cases miscarriage occurs at the fifth or seventh month, and if the children are
born alive they rarely survive long. Lead exerts a similar influence on the reproductive powers in the male sex; men with lead
affections seldom produce healthy children." Many of these dis-

eases might be prevented, if the excessive number of workers did not make the prevention a matter of indifference to those concerned. Dr. Thompson says: "Let over-crowding and over-heating be avoided. There should be an abundant supply of pure air. The hours of work should be moderate, with fair intervals for meals. If there is much dust or other foreign matter in the air a suitable respirator should be used, or the offensive particles should be carried off by a current of air produced by a chimney or revolving wheel. Again, mechanical appliances may often take the place of hand-labor, and much may often be accomplished by the application of practical science and chemical knowledge." Thus we see indifference to life resulting from the over-crowding of the labor market, and in the unhealthy conditions among which many kinds of work are carried on we find a widely-spread check to population.

Baby-farming has only too justly been called the "hideous social phaenomenon of the nineteenth century." It is the direct result of the pressure of over-large families, and is simply a veiled form of infanticide. Mr. Benson Baker, one of the medical officers of Marylebone, has written a sad notice of baby-farming. He speaks of a notorious case: "One of the stock from that model baby-farm is now under my care. This child, three years old, was employed by the proprietress as a gaffer or ganger over the younger babies. His duties were to sit up in the middle of the bed with eight other babies round him, and the moment any one of them awoke to put the bottle to their mouth. He was also to keep them quiet, and generally to superintend them." A vast number of children are slowly murdered annually in this way, and the death-rate is also very high in every place where many infants are kept together, whether it be in workhouse, hospital, or crèche.

Another consequence of large families which must not be overlooked is the physical injury caused to the mothers. Among the poor, cases of *prolapsus uteri,* or falling of the womb, are only too common; *prolapsus uteri* results frequently from "getting about" too rapidly after child-birth, it being impossible for the mother of the increasing family to lie by for that period of rest which nature absolutely enjoins. "Women," says Dr. Drysdale, "ought never to get up from confinement for some weeks after the child is born; but these poor women are so utterly unable to do without work that they are compelled to get up in a day or two. The womb being full of blood, falls down and produces infirmity for life." The doctor also says of this disease: "It is extremely common. Indeed, when I was obstetrical assistant at Edinburgh, it was one of the commonest diseases among women—the principal one, in fact." "Prolapsus, or falling of the womb," says Dr. Graily Hewett, "is an affection to which women are in one form or other exceedingly liable, and it is one which is not unfrequently productive of very much inconvenience and distress." The reason of the disease is not far to see. The womb, in its unimpregnated state, is "from two and a half to three inches long, and an inch and a half wide, more or less, at its largest part, and about an inch thick" (Dr. Marion Sims). During the nine months of pregnancy this organ is stretched more and more, until, at the end of nine months, it is capable of containing the fully developed infant. During these nine months the muscular substance of the womb "increases in thickness, while the whole organ enlarges in order to accommodate the growing foetus and its appendages" (Dr. Dalton). At birth the muscular fibres begin to contract, and the womb ought to return to almost its original size. But in order that it may so return, the horizontal position is absolutely necessary for some days, and much rest for some weeks, until the muscles connected with the womb have regained something of their natural elasticity. If the mother be forced to leave her bed too early, if she be compelled to exert herself in housekeeping cares, to stand over the washtub, to bend over the fire—what happens? The womb, so long distended, has no chance of healthy contraction; the muscles which support it in its proper position have not recovered from the long strain; the womb itself is heavy with the blood flowing from the vessels yet unclosed, and it naturally falls and "produces infirmity for life." Too frequent pregnancy is another cause of *prolapsus uteri,* and of many other diseases of the womb. "We frequently find that the uterus becomes diseased from the fact that the pregnancies rapidly succeed each other, the uterus not having recovered its natural size when it becomes again occupied by an ovum" (Dr. Graily Hewett). The womb is too constantly put on the stretch, and is not allowed sufficient rest to recover its original vigor and elasticity. It takes about two months for the womb to thoroughly reconstruct itself after the delivery of a child; a new mucous membrane develops, and a degeneration and reconstruction of the muscles takes place, technically known as "the involution of the uterus." During pregnancy, the uterine muscles "increase very considerably in size. Their texture becomes much more distinctly granular, and their outlines more strongly marked. . . . The entire walls of the uterus, at the time of delivery, are composed of such muscular fibres, arranged in circular, oblique, and longitudinal bundles. About the end of the first week after delivery, these fibres begin to undergo a fatty degeneration. . . . The muscular fibers which have become altered by the fatty deposit, are afterwards gradually absorbed and disappear, their place being subsequently taken by other fibres of new formation, which already begin to make their appearance before the old ones have been completely destroyed. As this process goes on, it results finally in a complete renovation of the muscular substance of the uterus. The organ becomes again reduced in size, compact in tissue, and of a pale ruddy hue, as in the ordinary unimpregnated condition. This entire renewal or reconstruction of the uterus is completed, according to Heschl, about the end of the second month after delivery" (Dr. Dalton). No words can add strength to this statement, proving the absolute right of women to complete repose from sexual disturbance during this slow recovery of the normal condition of the womb. Many a woman in fairly comfortable circumstances suffers from lack of knowledge of physical laws, and from the reckless English disregard of all conjugal prudence. Short of absolute displacement of the womb, and of grave uterine diseases, various disorders result from weakness of the over-taxed generative organs. Leucorrhea is one of the commonest of these, producing general debility, pain in the back, indigestion, &c. It is not right, it is not moral, that mothers of families should thus ruin their health, causing suffering to themselves and misery to those around them; it is only a perverted moral sense which leads men and women to shut their eyes to these sad consequences of over-large families, and causes them thus to disregard the plainest laws of health. Sexual intemperance, the over-procreation of children, is as immoral as intemperance in drink.

Among the melancholy consequences of over-population we must not omit the foolish and sometimes criminal attempts made by ignorant people to limit the family; the foolish attempt is the prevalent habit of over-lactation, arising from the mistaken idea that conception is impossible during the nursing of a child; the criminal attempt is the procuring of abortion by means of drugs or by the use of instruments. These will be more fully dealt with in Chapter III, and are only alluded to here as among the consequences of the pressure of over-population. Too often, indeed, do these come under the head of the positive, the life-destroying checks.

To turn to a different and more immediately life-destroying class of checks, that of war cannot, of course, be left out of this melancholy picture. Great famines are positive checks on a still more frightful scale. Lord Derby says as to India: "If present appearances can be trusted, we shall have in every generation a larger aggregate of human beings relying upon us for help in those periods of distress which must from time to time occur in a country wholly agricultural and liable to droughts." But what a confession of helplessness! Is it possible to sit down with folded hands and calmly contemplate the recurrence at regular intervals of such a famine as lately slew its tens of thousands? Yet the law of population is "an irrefragable truth," and these people are starved to death according to natural law; early marriages, large families, these are the premises; famine and disease, these are the conclusions. The same consequences will, sooner or later—

sooner in an agricultural country, dependent on its crops, later in a manufacturing country commanding large foreign supplies, but always inexorably—produce the same fearful results.

One more melancholy positive check must be added, the last to which we shall here refer. It is the absolute child-murder by desertion or by more violent means: Dr. Lankester said that "there were in London alone 16,000 women who had murdered their offspring." Dr. Attwood lately stated of Macclesfield that the doctors in that town often had moral, though not legal, proof that children were "put away," and that Macclesfield was "no worse than any other manufacturing town."

Such are some of the consequences of the law of population; the power of production is held in check by the continual destruction, the number of births is balanced by the number of deaths. Population struggles to increase, but the want of the means of existence beats it back, and men, women, and children perish in the terrible struggle. The more civilisation advances the more hopeless becomes the outlook. The checks imposed by "nature and providence," in which Sir Hardinge Gifford trusts for the prevention of over-population, are being removed, one by one, by science and by civilisation. War will be replaced by arbitration, and those who would have fallen victims to it will become fathers of families; sanitary knowledge will bring sanitary improvement, and typhus fever and smallpox will disappear as the plague and black death have done; children will not die in their infancy, and the average length of human life will increase. The life-destroying checks of "nature and providence" will be met with the life-preserving attempts of science and of reason, and population will increase more and more rapidly. What will be the result? Simply this: India to-day is a microcosm of the world of the future, and the statesman of that time will re-echo the words of the present Foreign Secretary with a wider application. Ought we then to encourage positive checks so as to avert this final catastrophe? Ought we to stir up war? Ought we to prevent sanitary improvements? Ought we to leave the sickly to die? Ought we to permit infants to perish unaided? Ought we to refuse help to the starving? These checks may be "natural," but they are not human; they may be "providential," but they are not rational. Has science no help for us in our extremity? has reason no solution to this problem? has thought no message of salvation to the poor?

CHAPTER III

## Its Bearing Upon Human Conduct and Morals

To THE question that closes the last chapter there *is* an answer; all thinkers have seen that since population increases more rapidly than the means of subsistence, the human brain should be called in to devise a restriction of the population, and so relieve man from the pressure of the struggle for existence. The lower animals are helpless, and must needs suffer, and strive, and die, but man, whose brain raises him above the rest of animated existence, man rational, thoughtful, civilised, he is not condemned to share in the brute struggle, and to permit lower nature to destroy his happiness and his ever-growing rapidity of progress. In dealing with the law of population, as with every other natural law which presses on him unpleasantly, civilised man seeks so to alter the conditions which surround him as to produce a happier result. Thinkers have, therefore, studied the law and its consequences, and have suggested various views of its bearing on human conduct and morals. It was acknowledged that the only way of escape from pauperism and from the misery occasioned by positive checks, was in the limitation of the population within the available means of subsistence, and the problem to be solved was—How shall this be done? Malthus proposed that preventive, or birth-restricting, should be substituted for positive, or life-destroying, checks, and that "moral restraint" should supersede "misery and vice." He lays it down as a principle of duty, that no one "is to bring beings into the world for whom he cannot find the means of support." This obligation, he says, is a "duty intelligible to the humblest capacity."

But the duty being admitted on all sides, the crucial point is— How is this duty to be fulfilled? Malthus answers:—By delay of marriage. We are bound "not to marry till we have a fair prospect of being able to support our children;" in a right state of society "no man, whose earnings were only sufficient to maintain two children, would put himself in a situation in which he might have to maintain four or five;" a man should "defer marrying, till, by industry and economy, he is in a capacity to support the children that he may reasonably expect from his marriage." Thus marriage—if ever possible to the poor—would be delayed until the middle of life, and the birth-rate would be decreased by a general abstention from marriage until a comparatively late age.

This preventive check would doubtless be an effectual one, but it is open to grave and fatal objections, and would only replace one set of evils by another. If late marriage were generally practised the most melancholy results would follow. The more marriage is delayed, the more prostitution spreads. It is necessary to gravely remind all advocates of late marriage that men do not and will not live single; and all women, and all men who honor women, should protest against a teaching which would inevitably make permanent that terrible social evil which is the curse of civilisation, and which condemns numbers of unhappy creatures to a disgraceful and revolting calling. Prostitution is an evil which we should strive to eradicate, not to perpetuate, and late marriage, generally adopted, would most certainly perpetuate it. The state of the streets of our large towns at nightfall is the result of deferred marriage, and marriage is deferred owing to the ever-increasing difficulty of maintaining a large family in anything like comfort.

Mr. Montagu Cookson, writing in the *Fortnightly Review,* says: "If, indeed, we could all become perfect beings, the rule of life deduced by Malthus from the unalterable law of population would be both practicable and safe; as it is, it has a direct tendency to promote the cardinal vice of cities—that of unchastity. The number of women in England who ply the loathsome trade of prostitution is already large enough to people a county, and, as our great thoroughfares show at nightfall, is certainly not diminishing. Their chief supporters justify themselves by the very plea which Malthus uses to enforce the duty of continence, namely, that they are not well enough off to maintain a wife and family. If they could be sure that they could limit the number of their children, so as to make it commensurate with their income, not only would the plea be generally groundless, but I believe it would not be urged, and the so-called social evil would be stormed in its strongest fortress."

The evils resulting from late marriage to those who remain really celibate, must not be overlooked in weighing this recommendation of it as a cure for the evils of over-population. Celibacy is not natural to men or to women; all bodily needs require their legitimate satisfaction, and celibacy is a disregard of natural law. The asceticism which despises the body is a contempt of nature, and a revolt against her; the morality which upholds virginity as the type of womanly perfection is unnatural; to be in harmony with nature, men and women should be husbands and wives, fathers and mothers, and until nature evolves a neuter sex celibacy will ever be a mark of imperfection. Very clearly has nature marked celibacy with disapproval; the average life of the unmarried is shorter than the average life of the married; the unmarried have a less vigorous physique, are more withered, more rapidly aged, more peevish, more fanciful; "the disordered emotions of persons of both sexes who pass lives of voluntary or enforced celibacy," says Dr. Drysdale in his essay on Prostitution, "is a fact of every-day observation. Their bad temper, fretfulness, and excitability are proverbial." We quote from the same tractate the following opinions: "M. Villamay, in his 'Dictionnaire des Sciences Médicales,' says: 'It is assuredly true that absolute and involuntary abstinence is the most common cause of hysteria.' Again, at a meeting of the Medico-Chirurgical Society, reported in the *Lancet* of February 14th, 1859, Mr. Holmes Coote is reported to have said: 'No doubt incontinence was a great sin; but the evils connected with continence were productive of far greater misery to society. Any person could bear witness to this, who had had experience in the wards of lunatic asylums.' Again, Sir Benjamin Brodie, at the Birmingham Social Science Meeting, is reported to have said, in a discussion on prostitution, that 'the evils of celibacy were so great that he would not mention them; but that they quite equalled those of prostitution!' " M. Block informs us that in France, out of 100 male lunatics, 65.72 are celibate, 5.61 are widowers, and only 28.67 are married; of 100 female lunatics, 58.16 are celibate; 12.48 are widows, and 29.36 are married. M. Bertillon, dealing with France, Holland, and Belgium, states that men who live celibate lives after twenty have, on an average, six years less of life than those who marry. The same fact holds good as regards married and unmarried women. A long train of formidable diseases results from celibacy—such as spermatorrhoea in the male, chlorosis and hysteria in the female—and no one who desires society to be happy and healthy should recommend late marriage as a cure for the social evils around us. Early marriage is best, both physically and morally; it guards purity, softens the affections, trains the heart, and preserves physical health; it teaches thought for others, gentleness and self-control; it makes men gentler and women braver from the contact of their differing natures. The children that spring from such marriages— where not following each other too rapidly—are more vigorous and healthy than those born of middle-aged parents, and in the ordinary course of nature the parents of such children live long enough to see them make their start in life, to aid, strengthen, and counsel them at the beginning of their career.

Fortunately, late marriage will never be generally practised in any community; the majority of men and women will never consent to remain single during the brightness of youth, when passion is strongest and feelings most powerful, and to marry only when life is half over and its bloom and its beauty have faded into middle-age. But it is important that late marriage should not even be regarded as desirable, for if it became an accepted doctrine among the thoughtful that late marriage was the only escape from over-population, a serious difficulty would arise; the best of the people, the most careful, the most provident, the most intelligent, would remain celibate and barren, while the careless, thoughtless, thriftless ones would marry and produce large families. This evil is found to prevail to some extent even now; the more thoughtful, seeing the misery resulting from large families on low wage, often abstain from marriage, and have to pay heavy poor-rates for the support of the thoughtless and their families, The preventive check proposed by Malthus must therefore be rejected, and a wiser solution of the problem must be sought.

Later thinkers, recognising at once the evils of over-population and the evils of late marriage, have striven to find a path which shall avoid both Scylla and Charybdis, and have advocated early marriages and small families. John Stuart Mill has been one of the most earnest of these true friends of the people; in his "Political Economy" he writes: "In a very backward state of society, like that of Europe in the Middle Ages, and many parts of Asia at present, population is kept down by actual starvation.... In a more improved state, few, even among the poorest of the people, are limited to actual necessaries, and to a bare sufficiency of those; and the increase is kept within bounds, not by excess of deaths, but by limitation of births. The limitation is brought about in various ways. In some countries, it is the result of prudent or conscientious self-restraint. There is a condition to which the laboring people are habituated; they perceive that by having too numerous families they must sink below that condition, or fail to transmit it to their children; and this they do not choose to submit to. The countries in which, so far as is known, a great degree of voluntary prudence has been longest practised on this subject are Norway and parts of Switzerland.... In both these countries the increase of population is very slow; and what checks it is not multitude of deaths, but fewness of births. Both the births and the deaths are remarkably few in proportion to the population; the average duration of life is the longest in Europe; the population contains fewer children, and a greater proportional number of persons in the vigor of life than is known to be the case in any other part of the world. The paucity of births tends directly to prolong life, by keeping the people in comfortable circumstances." Clearly and pointedly

Mill teaches "conjugal prudence;" he quotes with approval the words of Sismondi, who was "among the most benevolent of his time, and the happiness of whose married life has been celebrated:" "When dangerous prejudices have not become accredited, when a morality contrary to our true duties towards others, and especially towards those to whom we have given life, is not inculcated in the name of the most sacred authority, no prudent man contracts matrimony before he is in a condition which gives him an assured means of living, and no married man has a greater number of children than he can properly bring up." Many other eminent men and women have spoken in the same sense; Professor Leone Levi advocates "prudence as regards the increase of our families." Mrs. Fawcett writes: "Those who deal with this question of pauperism should remember that it is not to be remedied by cheap food, by reductions of taxation, or by economical administration in the departments, or by new forms of government. Nothing will permanently affect pauperism while the present reckless increase of population continues." Mr. Montagu Cookson says that some may think "prudential restraint after marriage wilder than anything Malthus ever dreamt," but urges that "the numbers of children born after marriage should be limited," and that "such limitation is as much the duty of married persons as the observance of chastity is the duty of those that are unmarried."

It remains, then, to ask how is this duty to be performed? It is clearly useless to preach the limitation of the family and to conceal the means whereby such limitation may be effected. If the limitation be a duty it cannot be wrong to afford such information as shall enable people to discharge it.

There are various prudential checks which have been suggested, but further investigation of this intricate subject is sorely needed, and it is much to be wished that more medical men would devote themselves to the study of this important branch of physiology. At present all one can do is to lay before the public the various checks suggested, on every one of which controversy is rife.

The check we will take first in order is that to which Mr.

Montagu Cookson alludes in his essay; he says that the family may be limited by "obedience to natural laws which all may discover and verify if they will." The "natural laws" to which Mr. Cookson refers, would be, we imagine, the results of observation on the comparative fertility with women of some periods over others. It is well known that the menstrual discharge, or the Catamenia, recurs in normal cases at monthly intervals, during the whole of the fertile period of female life; a woman does not bear children before menstruation has commenced, nor after it has ceased. There are cases on record where women have borne children but have never menstruated, but these are rare exceptions to the general rule; menstruation is the sign of capability of conception, as its cessation is the sign of future disability to conceive. Recent investigators have collected many cases in which "the menstrual period was evidently connected with the maturation and discharge of ova" (Carpenter). "The essential part of the female generative system," says Dr. Carpenter, "is that in which the ova (eggs) are prepared. . . . In the higher animals, as in the human female, the substance of the ovarium is firm and compact, and consists of a nucleated, tough, fibrous, connective tissue, with much interspersed fusiform muscular tissue, forming what is known as the *stroma*. . . . As development proceeds the cells . . . multiply, and single cells or groups of cells, round, ovoid, or tubular, come to be enclosed in the tissue of the ovary by delicate vascular processes which shoot forth from the stroma. These cells constitute the primordial ova." These ova gradually mature, and are then discharged from the ovary and pass into the uterus, and on the fertilisation of one of them conception depends. Dr. Kirke writes: "It has long been known that in the so-called oviparous animals the separation of ova from the ovary may take place independently of impregnation by the male, or even of sexual union. And it is now established that a like maturation and discharge of ova, independently of coition, occurs in mammalia, the periods at which the matured ova are separated from the ovaries and received into the Fallopian tubes being indicated in the lower mammalia by the phaenomena of *heat* or *rut;* in the human female by the phaenomena of *menstrua-*

*tion*. . . . It may, therefore, be concluded that the two states, heat and menstruation, are analogous, and that the essential accompaniment of both is the maturation and extrusion of ova." Seeing, then, that the ova are discharged at the menstrual period, and that conception depends on the fertilisation of the ova by the male, it is obvious that conception will most readily take place immediately before or after menstruation. "It is quite certain that there is a greater aptitude for conception immediately before and after that epoch than there is at any intermediate period" (Carpenter). A woman "is more apt to conceive soon after menstruation than at any other time" (Chavasse). So much is this fact recognised by the medical profession, that in cases of sterility a husband is often recommended only to visit his wife immediately after the cessation of the Catamenia. Since women conceive more easily at this period, the avoidance of sexual intercourse during the few days before and after menstruation has been recommended as a preventive check. Dr. Tyler Smith writes: "In the middle of the interval between the periods, there is little chance of impregnation taking place. The same kind of knowledge is of use, by way of caution, to women who menstruate during lactation, in whom there is a great aptitude to conceive; pregnancy, under such circumstances, would be injurious to the health of the foetus, the child at the breast, and the mother herself, and therefore should be avoided, if possible." The most serious objection to reliance on this check is that it is not certain. M. Raciborski says that only six or seven per cent of conceptions take place during this interval, but the six or seven exceptions to the general rule prevent recommendation of the check as thoroughly reliable; we can scarcely say more than that women are far less likely to conceive midway between the menstrual periods than either immediately before or after them.

The preventive check advocated by Dr. Knowlton consists in the use of the ordinary syringe immediately after intercourse, a solution of sulphate of zinc or of alum being used instead of water. It is probable that this check is an effective one, a most melancholy proof of its effectiveness being given by Dr. J. C. Barr, who, giving evidence before the Commission on the working of the Contagious Diseases Act, stated: "Every woman who leaves the hospital is instructed in the best mode of preventing disease. These are cleanliness, injections of alum, and sulphate of zinc." Professor Sheldon Amos, dealing with the same painful subject, refers to this evidence, and quotes Dr. Barr, as saying again: "My custom is to instruct them to keep themselves clean, to use injections and lotions." These women are not meant to bear children, they are to be kept "fit for use" by Her Majesty's soldiers. Apart altogether from this sad, but governmentally authorised, use of this check, there are many obvious disadvantages connected with it as a matter of taste and feeling.

The check which appears to us to be preferable, as grating on no feeling of affection or of delicacy, is that recommended by Carlile many years ago in his "Every Woman's Book." In order that impregnation should take place, "the absolute contact of the spermatozoa with the ovum is requisite" (Carpenter). The ovum passes from the ovary down the Fallopian tube into the uterus; the spermatazoa, floating in the spermatic fluid, pass upwards through the uterus, and fecundate the ovum either in the uterus, in the tube, or in the ovary itself. To prevent impregnation it is then only necessary to prevent this contact. The neck of the uterus, where it enters the vagina, ends with the *Os uteri,* an orifice varying in shape in different individuals. Through this orifice the male semen must pass in order to fertilise the ovum. To prevent impregnation, pass to the end of the vagina a piece of fine sponge, which should be dipped in water before being used, and which need not be removed until the morning. Dr. Marion Sims, who in cases of retroversion of the uterus constantly used mechanical support to maintain the uterus in its normal position, and so make pregnancy possible, gives much useful information on the various kinds of pessaries. He sometimes used a "small wad of cotton, not more than an inch in diameter," which was "secured with a string for its removal;" this was worn during the day and removed at night. He says that the woman using a pessary should be able "to remove and replace it with the same facility that she would put on and pull off an old slipper." There is, in fact, no kind of difficulty in the use of this check, and it has the great advantage of unobtrusiveness.

There is a preventive check attempted by many poor women which is most detrimental to health, and should therefore never be employed, namely the too-long persistence in nursing one baby, in the hope of thereby preventing the conception of another. *Nursing does not prevent conception.* A child should not be nursed, according to Dr. Chavasse, for longer than nine months; and he quotes Dr. Farr, as follows: "It is generally recognised that the healthiest children are those weaned at nine months complete. Prolonged nursing hurts both child and mother: in the child, causing a tendency to brain disease, probably through disordered digestion and nutrition; in the mother, causing a strong tendency to deafness and blindness." Dr. Chavasse adds: "If he be suckled after he be twelve months old, he is generally pale, flabby, unhealthy, and rickety; and the mother is usually nervous, emaciated, and hysterical. . . . A child nursed beyond twelve months is very apt, if he should live, to be knock-kneed, and bow-legged, and weak-ankled, to be narrow-chested, and chicken-breasted." If pregnancy occur, and the mother be nursing, the consequences affect alike the mother, the babe, and the unborn child. To nurse under these circumstances, says Dr. Chavasse, "is highly improper, and it not only injures her own health, and may bring on a miscarriage, but it is also prejudicial to her babe, and may produce a delicacy of constitution from which he might never recover."

Another class of checks is distinctly criminal, *i.e.,* the procuring of abortion. Various drugs are taken by women with this intent, and too often their use results in death, or in dangerous sickness. Dr. Fleetwood Churchill gives various methods of inducing labor prematurely, and argues, justly, that where the delivery of a living child at the full time is impossible, it is better to bring on labor than be compelled to perform later either craniotomy or the Caesarian section. But he goes further: "There are cases where the distortion [of the pelvis] is so great as to render the passage of a seven months' child impossible, and others still

THE LAW OF POPULATION

worse, where no reduction of the viable child's bulk will enable it to pass. I do not see why abortion should not be induced at an early stage in such cases." And Dr. Churchill quotes Mr. Ingleby as saying: "Premature labor may with great propriety be proposed on pregnancy recurring, assuming the delivery of a living child at term to have already proved impracticable." If there is a chance for the child's life, this is sound advice, but if the delivery of a living child has been proved to be impossible, surely the prevention of conception is far better than the procuring of abortion. The destruction of the foetus is destruction of life, and it is immoral, where a woman cannot bear a living child, that she should conceive at all.

If this system of preventive checks were generally adopted, how happy would be the result both to the home and to the State! The root of poverty would be dug up, and pauperism would decline and at last vanish. Where now overcrowded hovels stand would then be comfortable houses; where now the large family starves in rags, the small family would then live on sufficient food, clad in decent raiment; education would replace ignorance, and self-reliance would supersede charity. Where the work-house now frowns the busy school would then smile, and care and forethought for the then valuable lives would diminish the dangers of factory and of work-room. Prostitution would cease to flaunt in our streets, and the sacred home would be early built and joyously dwelt in; wedded love would enter the lists against vice, and, no longer the herald of want, would chase her counterfeit from our land. No longer would transmitted diseases poison our youth, nor premature death destroy our citizens. A full possibility of life would open before each infant born into our nation, and there would be room, and love, and cherishing enough for each new-comer. It remains for England to have all this if she will; but the first upward step towards that happier life will only be taken when parents resolutely determine to limit their family to their means, and stamp with moral disapprobation every married couple who selfishly overcrowd their home, to the injury of the community of which they are a part.

## CHAPTER IV

## Objections Considered

MANY people, perfectly good-hearted, but somewhat narrow-minded, object strongly to the idea of conjugal prudence, and regard scientific checks to population as "a violation of nature's laws, and a frustration of nature's ends." Such people, a hundred years ago, would have applauded the priest who objected to lightning conductors as being an interference with the bolts of Deity; they exist in every age, the rejoicers over past successes, and the timid disapprovers of new discoveries. Let us analyse the argument. "A violation of nature's laws;" this objection is couched in somewhat unscientific phrase; nature's "laws" are but the observed sequences of events; man cannot violate them; he may disregard them, and suffer in consequence; he may observe them, and regulate his conduct so as to be in harmony with them. Man's prerogative is that by the use of his reason he is able to study nature outside himself, and by observation may so control nature as to make her add to his happiness instead of bringing him misery. To limit the family is no more a violation of nature's laws than to preserve the sick by medical skill; the restriction of the birth-rate does not violate nature's laws more than does the restriction of the death-rate. Science strives to diminish the positive checks; science should also discover the best preventive checks. "The frustration of nature's ends." Why should we worship nature's ends? Nature flings lightning at our houses; we frustrate her ends by the lightning conductor. Nature divides us by seas and by rivers; we frustrate her ends by sailing over the seas, and by bridging the rivers. Nature sends typhus fever and ague to slay us; we frustrate her ends by purifying the air, and by draining the marshes. Oh! it is answered, you only do this by using other natural powers. Yes, we answer, and we only teach conjugal prudence by balancing one natural force against another. Such study of nature, and such balancing of natural forces, is civilisation.

It is next objected that preventive checks are "unnatural" and "immoral." "Unnatural" they are not; for the human brain is nature's highest product, and all improvements on irrational nature are most purely natural; preventive checks are no more unnatural than every other custom of civilisation. Raw meat, nakedness, living in caves, these are the *irrational* natural habits; cooked food, clothes, houses, these are the *rational* natural customs. Production of offspring recklessly, carelessly, lustfully, this is irrational nature, and every brute can here outdo us; production of offspring with forethought, earnestness, providence, this is rational nature, where man stands alone. But "immoral." What is morality? It is the greatest good of the greatest number. It is immoral to give life where you cannot support it. It is immoral to bring children into the world when you cannot clothe, feed, and educate them. It is immoral to crowd new life into already over-crowded houses, and to give birth to children wholesale, who never have a chance of healthy life. Conjugal prudence is most highly moral, and "those who endeavor to vilify and degrade these means in the eyes of the public, and who speak of them as 'immoral' and 'disgusting,' are little aware of the moral responsibility they incur thereby. As already shown, to reject preventive intercourse is in reality to choose the other three true population checks—poverty, prostitution, and celibacy. So far from meriting reprobation, the endeavor to spread the knowledge of the preventive methods, of the great law of nature which renders them necessary, is in my opinion the very greatest service which can at present be done to mankind" ("Elements of Social Science").

But the knowledge of these scientific checks would, it is argued, make vice bolder, and would increase unchastity among women by making it safe. Suppose that this were so, it might save some broken hearts and some deserted children; men ruin women and go scatheless, and then bitterly object that their victims escape something of public shame. And if so, are all to suffer, so that one or two already corrupt in heart may be preserved from becoming corrupt in act? Are mothers to die slowly that impure women may be held back, and wives to be sacrificed, that the unchaste may be curbed? As well say that no knives must be used because throats may be cut with them; no matches sold because incendiarism may result from them; no pistols allowed because murders may be committed by them. Blank ignorance has some advantages in the way of safety, and if all men's eyes were put out none would ever be tempted to seduce a woman for her beauty. Let us bring for our women the veil to cover and the eunuch to guard, and so be at least consistent in our folly and our distrust! But this knowledge would *not* increase unchastity; the women who could thus use it would be solely those who only lack opportunity, not will, to go astray; the means suggested all imply deliberation and forethought. Are these generally the handmaids of unchastity? English women are not yet sunk so low that they preserve their loyalty to one only from fear of the possible consequences of disloyalty; their purity, their pride, their honor, their womanhood, these are the guardians of their virtue, and never from English women's heart will fade the maiden and matronly dignity which makes them shield their love from all taint of impurity, and bid them only surrender themselves where the surrender of heart and of pledged faith have led the way. Shame on those who slander England's wives and maidens with the foul thoughts that can only spring from the mind and the lips of the profligate!

Another class of objectors appears—those who argue that there is no need to limit the population; at any rate for a long while to come. Some of these say that there is food enough in the world for all, and point out that the valley of the Mississippi would grow corn enough to feed the present population of the globe. They forget that the *available* means of subsistence are those with which we have to deal. Corn in Nebraska and starving mouths in Lancashire are not much use to each other. When the cost of carriage exceeds the money-power of the would-be buyer, the corn-fields might be in the moon for all the good they are to him. If means can be discovered of bringing corn and mouths together, well and good; but until they are discovered, undue production of mouths here is unwise, because their owners will starve while the corn is still on the other side of the sea.

But if the corn can't be brought to the mouths, may not the mouths go to the corn? Why not emigrate? Because emigration is impracticable to the extent needed for the relief of the labor market. Emigration caused by starvation pressure is not a healthy outlet for labor. If it is Government-aided, helpless, thriftless folk flock to it for a while, and starve on the other side. If land is given, capital is wanted by the emigrant, for before he can eat his own bread he must clear his land of timber, plough or dig it, sow his corn, and wait for his harvest. If he goes out poor on what is he to live during the first year? Men with £300 or £400 of capital may find more profitable investment for it in the West in America, or in our colonies, than at home; but their outgoing will not much relieve the labor market. Emigration for penniless agricultural laborers and for artisans means only starvation abroad instead of at home. And it is starvation under worse conditions than they had left in the mother-country. They have to face vicissitudes of climate for which they are utterly unprepared, extremes of heat and of cold which try even vigorous constitutions, and simply kill off underfed, half-clothed, and ill-housed new comers. Nor is work always to be had in the New World. No better proof of the foolishness of emigration to the United States can be given than the fact that at the present time contractors in England are in treaty with American workmen with the object of bringing them over here. Unskilled labor does not improve its chances by going abroad. Nor is skilled labor in a better position, for here the German emigrant undersells the British; he can live harder and cheaper, and has had a better technical education than has fallen to the lot of his British rival. One great evil connected with emigration is the disproportion it causes between men and women, both in the old country and in the new, those who emigrate being chiefly males. Nor must it be forgotten that when England colonised most, her population was far smaller than it is at the present time. Physical vigor is necessary for successful colonising, and the physical vigor of our laboring poor deteriorates under their present conditions. As the

Canadian roughly said at the meeting of the British Association at Plymouth: "The colonies don't want the children of your rickety paupers." Colonisation needs the pick of a nation, if it is to succeed, not the poor who are driven from home in search of the necessaries of life. John Stuart Mill points out how inadequate emigration is as a continued relief to population, useful as it is as a sudden effort to lighten pressure. He remarks that the great distance of the fields of emigration prevents them from being a sufficient outlet for surplus laborers; "it still remains to be shown by experience," he says, "whether a permanent stream of emigration can be kept up sufficient to take off, as in America, all that portion of the annual increase (when proceeding at its greatest rapidity) which, being in excess of the progress made during the same short period in the arts of life, tends to render living more difficult for every averagely situated individual in the community. And unless this can be done, emigration cannot, even in an economical point of view, dispense with the necessity of checks to population." 1,173 infants are born in the United Kingdom every day, and to equalise matters about 1,000 emigrants should leave our shores daily. Careful calculations are sometimes entered into by anti-Malthusians as to the acreage of Great Britain as compared with its population, and it is said that the land would support many more than the present number of inhabitants; quite so; there is a very large quantity of land used for deer, game, and pleasure, that, if put under cultivation, would enormously increase the food-supply. But to know this, does not remedy the pressing evils of over-population; what service is it to the family crowded into a St. Giles' cellar to tell them that there are large uninhabited tracts of land in Perthshire? In the first place they can't get to them, and if they could, they would be taken up for trespassing. Such information is but mockery. Land reform is sorely needed, but, to meet the immediate needs of the present, land revolution would be necessary; it is surely wiser to lessen the population-pressure, and to work steadily at the same time towards Reform of the Land Laws, instead of allowing the population-pressure to increase, until the starving multitudes precipitate us into a revolution.

An extraordinary confusion exists in some minds between

preventive checks and infanticide. People speak as though prevention were the same as destruction. But no life is destroyed by the prevention of conception, any more than by abstention from marriage; if it is infanticide for every man and woman not to produce as many children as possible during the fertile period of life, if every person in a state of celibacy commits infanticide because of the potential life he prevents, then, of course, the prevention of conception by married persons is also infanticide; the two things are on exactly the same level. When conception has taken place, then prevention is no longer possible, and a new life having been made, the destruction of that life would be criminal. Before conception no life exists to be destroyed; the seminal fluid is simply a secretion of the body; its fertilising power is not a living thing, the non-use of which destroys life; the spermatozoa, the active fertilising agents, are not living existences, and "they have been erroneously considered as proper animalculae" (Carpenter). Life is not made until the male and female elements are united, and if this is prevented, either by abstention from intercourse among the unmarried, or by preventive intercourse among the married, life is not destroyed, because the life is not yet in existence.

Mr. Darwin puts forward an argument against scientific checks which must not be omitted here; he says: "The enhancement of the welfare of mankind is a most intricate problem; all ought to refrain from marriage who cannot avoid abject poverty for their children, for poverty is not only a great evil, but tends to its own increase by leading to recklessness in marriage. On the other hand, as Mr. Galton has remarked, if the prudent avoid marriage, whilst the reckless marry, the inferior members tend to supplant the better members of society. Man, like every other animal, has no doubt advanced to his present high condition through a struggle for existence, consequent on his rapid multiplication, and if he is to advance still higher it is to be feared that he must remain subject to a severe struggle; otherwise he would sink into indolence, and the more gifted men would not be more successful in the battle of life than the less gifted. Hence our natural rate of increase, though leading to many and obvious evils, must not be greatly diminished by any means."

If the struggle for existence among mankind were waged under the same conditions as among animals, then Mr. Darwin's argument would have great force, terrible as would be the amount of human misery caused by it. Then the strongest, cleverest, craftiest, would survive, and would transmit their qualities to their offspring. But Mr. Darwin forgets that men have qualities which the brutes have not, such as compassion, justice, respect for the rights of others—and all these, man's highest virtues, are absolutely incompatible with the brutal struggle for existence. Where the lion would leave his parents to starve, man would feed his; where the stag would kill the sickly one, man would carry him to the hospital and nurse him back to health. The feeble, the deformed, the helpless are killed out in brute nature; in human nature they are guarded, tended, nourished, and they hand on to their offspring their own disabilities. Scientific checks to population would just do for man what the struggle for existence does for the brutes: they enable man to control the production of new human beings; those who suffer from hereditary diseases, who have consumption or insanity in the family, might marry, if they so wished, but would preserve the race from the deterioration which results from propagating disease. The whole British race would gain in vigor, in health, in longevity, in beauty, if only healthy parents gave birth to children; at present there is many a sickly family, because sickly persons marry; they revolt against forbiddance of marriage, celibacy being unnatural, and they are taught that "the natural consequences of marriage" must follow. Let them understand that one set of "consequences" results naturally from one set of conditions, another set from different conditions, and let them know that *laisser aller* in marriage is no wiser than in other paths of life.

Leaving objectors let us look at the other side of the question. The system of preventive checks to population points us to the true pathway of safety; it is an immediate relief, and at once lightens the burden of poverty. Each married couple have it in their power to avoid poverty for themselves and for their children, by determining, when they enter on married life, that they will not produce a family larger than they can comfortably maintain: thus they avoid the daily harass of domestic struggle; they rejoice over two healthy, robust, well-fed children, instead of mourning over seven frail, sickly, half-starved ones; they look forward to an old age of comfort and of respectability instead of one of painful dependence on a grudgingly-given charity.

How rapidly conjugal prudence may lift a nation out of pauperism is seen in France; the proportion of adults to the whole population is the largest in Europe, the proportionate number of persons under thirty being the smallest; hence, there are more producers and fewer non-producers than in any other country. The consequence of this is that the producers are less pressed upon, and live in greater comfort and with more enjoyment of life. There are no less than 5,000,000 of properties under six acres, each sufficient to support a small family, but wholly inadequate for the maintenance of a large one, and it was from these independent peasants that M. Thiers borrowed the money to pay off the indemnity levied by the Germans after the late war. If those peasants had been struggling under the difficulties of large families, no savings would have been made to fall back upon in such an emergency. France shows a pattern of widely-spread comfort which we look for in vain in our own land, and this comfort is directly traceable to the systematic regard for conjugal prudence. Small agricultural holdings directly tend to this virtue, the fact of the limitation of the food-supply available being obvious to the most ignorant peasant. So strongly rooted is this habit in France that the Roman Church in vain branded it as a deadly sin, and Dr. Drysdale writes that a French priest begged the Vatican Council to change this direction; he said: "It is not the sin which is new, but the circumstances which have changed. This practice has been spreading more and more for half a century from the force of things. As Providence does not multiply animals, when they have not wherewithal to eat, so it will not require reasonable man voluntarily to multiply when there is no longer the condition for his subsistence. This is human calculation, pecuniary motives if you will, but a calculation as inevitable as destiny. Countries enjoying the faith do not thus calculate, it is true, and so long as obedience is possible they will obey the priest without a murmur; but a day will come when the prevailing doctrine will be applicable to them all, and hence we earnestly plead for reform. Other times, other customs. The laws should change with the customs."

It is well worthy of notice that those who have pleaded for scientific checks to population have also been those who have been identified with the struggle for political and religious freedom; Carlile defended the use of such—as advocated in his "Every Woman's Book"—as follows:—

"There are four grounds on which my 'Every Woman's Book' and its recommendation can be defended, and each of them in itself is sufficient to justify the publication, and to make it meritorious. First—the political or national ground; which refers to the strength and wealth of the nation, and the greatest happiness of the greatest number of the people. Second—the local or commercial ground, or the ground of the wages of labor, and its supply in the several trades and districts. Third—the domestic or family ground, where the parents may think they have already children enough, and that more will be an injury. Fourth—the individual ground, where the state of health in the female, or her situation in life, will not justify a pregnancy; but where the abstinence from love becomes as great an evil. . . . It is objected to me that there is a sufficiency of natural checks already in existence, to remedy the evils of which I complain. My answer is, that these natural checks are the evil of which I do complain, and *which I seek to remove by the substitution of a* MORAL CHECK, *that shall furnish no pain, no degradation; no discomfort, no evil of any kind.* The existing natural or physical checks are disease or pestilence and famine. Surely it is to be desired that neither of these should exist. It is not wise, not parental, not kind, to breed children to such disasters. It is better that they should not be born than be cut off prematurely by disease or famine, or struggle through a life of disease, poverty, and misery, a life of pain to themselves, and both a pain and burthen to their parents."

Mr. Francis Place argues: "The mass of the people in an old

country must remain in a state of wretchedness, until they are convinced that their safety depends upon themselves, and that it can be maintained in no other way than by their ceasing to propagate faster than the means of comfortable subsistence are produced.... If above all it were once clearly understood that it was not disreputable for married persons to avail themselves of such precautionary means as would, without being injurious to health, or destructive of female delicacy, *prevent conception,* a sufficient check might at once be given to the increase of population beyond the means of subsistence, and vice and misery to a prodigious extent might be removed from society."

Mr. James Watson showed his view of the matter by publishing Dr. Charles Knowlton's "Fruits of Philosophy."

Mr. Robert Dale Owen (son of Robert Owen, and American minister in Florence), in his "Moral Physiology," advocates and describes scientific checks.

Mr. James Mill says that "if the superstitions of the nursery were disregarded, and the principle of utility kept steadily in view, a solution might not be very difficult to be found."

Mr. John Stuart Mill strongly urges restraint of the number of the family, and he took an active part in disseminating the knowledge of scientific checks.

The members of the old Freethought Institution in John Street made it part of their work to circulate popular tracts, advocating scientific checks, such as a four-page tract entitled: "Population: is not its increase at present an evil, and would not some harmless check be desirable?"

Mr. Austin Holyoake, in his "Large and Small Families," follows in the same strain, and recommends as guides Knowlton's pamphlet and Owen's "Moral Physiology."

Mr. George Jacob Holyoake, writing as one of the Vice-Presidents of the National Secular Society in 1876, points to the difference between Christian and Secular morality on this head; he says: "Let any one regard for a moment the Christian's theory of this life. It tells us that all human beings born are immortal, and that God has to provide for them above or below! Yet in every portion of the land scoundrel or vicious parents may bring into

existence a squalid brood of dirty, sickly, depraved, ignorant, rag-
ged children. Christianity fails utterly to prevent their existence,
and hurls quick words of opprobrium upon any who advocate
the prevention of this progeny of crime. Yet the Christian
teaches that, by mere act of orthodox belief, these ignorant and
unclean creatures can be sent from the gutter to God. A Secularist cannot help shuddering at this doctrine and this practice,
so fatal to society, so contemptuous to heaven."

Thus has the effort to obtain social reform gone hand in hand
with that for political and religious freedom; the victors in the
latter have been the soldiers in the former. Discussion on the
Population Question is not yet safe; legal penalty threatens those
who advocate the restriction of birth instead of the destruction of
life; the same penalty was braved by our leaders in the last generation, and we have only to follow in their steps in order to
conquer as they conquered and become sharers of their crown.
We work for the redemption of the poor, for the salvation of the
wretched; the cause of the people is the sacredest of all causes,
and is the one which is the most certain to triumph however
sharp may be the struggle for the victory.

# THEOSOPHY AND

# THE LAW OF

# POPULATION

BY

ANNIE BESANT.

---

BENARES:

THEOSOPHICAL PUBLISHING SOCIETY.

LONDON:

THEOSOPHICAL PUBLISHING SOCIETY, 7, DUKE STREET, ADELPHI, W C

MADRAS:

THEOSOPHIST OFFICE, ADYAR.

---

1896.

---

*Price two Annas*

## Theosophy and the Law of Population

HUMAN lives may be builded on many foundations, but the life must always consist with the foundation if its conduct is to be orderly and coherent. In our social and political institutions we are wont to change our foundations and leave on them much of the old superstructures, heedless of the anachronisms perpetrated, as though a man were to walk about in frock coat and top hat with the bile and battle of his infancy tied round his neck. But the individual is on the whole, perhaps, more consistent than the community, lack of congruity being more glaring in the small organism than in the large. And it is certainly both wise and necessary to review opinions formed on one intellectual basis, if that basis is changed for another, since the logical and rightful outgrowth of the one may be illogical and wrong when translated to the other.

Twice, during my own intellectual life, I have changed the basis of my philosophy, on each occasion, as it seems to me, rising a step upwards on the side of the mountain on the summit of which stands the white Temple of Truth. Starting as a Christian, I accepted the ascetic and mystical side of Christianity, and had my dreams of treading in the steps of the saints and martyrs of the Church. Terrible was the price paid as purchase-money of intellectual freedom, the wrench from the old faith, the breaking with the beliefs that had made life sacred, and with the friends that had made it beautiful. Followed thereon the rebuilding of a theory of life on the basis of Materialism, the Judging of all by its effect on human happiness now and in future generations. The object of life became the ultimate building up of a physically, mentally, morally perfect man, by the cumulative effects of heredity, mental and moral tendencies being regarded as the outcome of material conditions, to be slowly but surely evolved by rational selection and the transmission to offspring of qualities carefully trained in and acquired by parents. The most characteristic note of this serious and lofty Materialism was struck by Professor W. Kingdon Clifford in his noble article on the "Ethics of Belief."

Taking this view of human duty to the race, it became of the first importance to rescue the control of the generation of offspring from mere blind brute passion, and to transfer it to the reason and intelligence; to impress on parents the sacredness of the parental office, the tremendous responsibility of the exercise of the creative function. And since, further, one of the most pressing problems for solution in the older countries is that of poverty, the horrible slums and dens into which are crowded and in which are festering families of eight and ten children, whose parents are earning an uncertain ten, twelve, fifteen, twenty shillings a week; since immediate palliative is wanted, if popular risings impelled by starvation are to be avoided; since the lives of men and women of the poorer classes and of the worst paid professional classes are one long heart-breaking struggle to "make both ends meet and keep respectable;" since in the middle-class, marriage is often avoided or delayed till late in life from the dread of a large family, and late marriage is followed by its shadow, the prevalence of vice and the moral and social ruin of thousands of women; for these, and many other reasons, the teaching of the duty of limiting the family within the means of subsistence is the logical outcome of Materialism. Seeking to improve the physical type, it would forbid parentage to any but healthy married couples, it would restrict child-bearing within the limits consistent with the thorough health and physical well-being of the mother; it would impose it as a duty never to bring children into the world unless the conditions for their Fair nurture and development are present; and regarding it as hopeless, as well as mischievous, to preach asceticism, and the conjunction of nominal celibacy with wide-spread prostitution as inevitable, from the constitution of human nature, it—quite rationally and logically—advises deliberate restriction of the production of offspring while sanctioning the exercise of the sexual instinct within the limits imposed by temperance, the highest physical and mental efficiency, the good order and dignity of society and the self-respect of the individual.

In all this there is nothing which for one moment implies approval of licentiousness, profligacy, unbridled self-indulgence. On the contrary, it is a well-considered and intellectually defensible scheme of human evolution, regarding all natural instincts as matters of regulation, not of destruction, and seeking to develop the perfectly healthy and well-balanced physical body as the necessary basis for the healthy and well-balanced mind. If the premisses of Materialism be true there is no answer to the neo-Malthusian conclusions, for even those Socialists who have bitterly opposed the promulgation of neo-Malthusianism regarding it as a "red herring intended to draw the attention of the proletariat away from the real cause of poverty, the monopoly of land and capital by a class"—admit that, when society is built on the foundation of common property in all that is necessary for the production of wealth, the time will come for the consideration of the population question. Apart from the Socialist antagonism, two main objections against neo-Malthusianism have been raised by thoughtful people as possibly valid. (1)—That it would lessen the struggle for existence, and so destroy the natural selection by which progress has been made in the past; (2) that only the more rational would adopt the theory, and so the production of offspring would diminish among the thoughtful while remaining as before among the ignorant and brutal, with the result that the population would be chiefly recruited from its baser instead of from its nobler elements. To the first objection the answer is that progress is made more rapidly and more economically by rational than by natural selection, and the time has arrived for man to control his own evolution instead of leaving it to the blind forces of nature. To the second, that already the least developed men and women are, as a rule, the most prolific, that high intellectual development is usually associated with a low rate of reproduction, and that we must face the inevitable; further, that the well-bred and carefully tended children of the thoughtful survive in much larger numbers than the neglected and poorly vitalised children of the vicious and the brutal, thus diminishing the original disproportion of numbers.

The famous trial of Mr. Charles Bradlaugh and myself for republishing a pamphlet on the subject written early in the century by Dr. Knowlton, an American physician, was the commencement of a great popular movement on the subject. We published the pamphlet because it was attacked by the police, and that did not seem to us the fashion in which such a question should be settled. We accordingly reprinted the tract, and sent notice to the police that we would personally sell them the pamphlet, so as to put no technical difficulties in the way of prosecution; we did so, and the trial was removed to the Court of Queen's Bench, on the writ of the Lord Chief Justice, who, after reading the pamphlet, decided that it was a scientific work, not an "obscene" one, in the ordinary sense of the word. To use his own phrase, it was a "dry physiological treatise." The prosecution was led by Sir Hardinge Gifford, the Solicitor General of the then Tory Government, who used every art of political and theological animosity against us; the judge, Sir Alexander Cockburn, Lord Chief Justice of England, was in strong sympathy with us, and summed up for us in a charge to the jury that was really a speech for the defence; the jury returned a special verdict completely exonerating us but condemning the book, and the judge reluctantly translated this into a verdict of Guilty. Obviously annoyed at the verdict he refused to give judgment, and let us go on our own recognisances. When we came up later for judgment, he urged us to surrender the pamphlet as the jury had condemned it; said our whole course with regard to it had been right, but that we ought to yield to the judgment of the jury. We were obstinate, and I shall never forget the pathetic way in which the great judge urged us to submit, and how at last, when we persisted that we would continue to sell it till the right to sell it was gained, he said that he would have let us go free if we would have yielded to the Court, but our persistence compelled him to sentence us. We gave notice of appeal, promising not to sell till the appeal was decided, and he let us go on our own recognisance. On appeal we quashed the verdict and went free;

we recoverd all the pamphlets seized and publicly sold them; we continued the sale till we received an intimation that no further prosecution would be attempted against us, and then dropped the sale of the pamphlet, and never took it up again. I wrote the "Law of Population" to replace it, and my pamphlet was never attacked, except in Australia, where the attack ignominiously failed, Justice Windeyer of the Supreme Court deciding in its favour in a remarkable judgment in which he justified the pamphlet and the neo-Malthusian position in one of the most luminous and cogent arguments I have ever read. The judgment was spoken of at the time in the English press as a "brilliant triumph for Mrs. Besant," and so I suppose it was; but no legal judgment could undo the harm wrought on the public mind by malignant and persistent misrepresentation in England. No one save myself will ever know what that trial cost me in pain: loss of children (through the judge said that my atheism alone justified their removal), loss of friends, social ostracism, with all the agony felt by a woman of pure life at being the butt of the vilest accusations. On the other hand there was the passionate gratitude evidenced by letters from thousands of poor married women—many from the wives of country clergymen and poor curates—thanking and blessing me for shewing them how to escape from the veritable hell in which they had lived. The "upper classes" of Society know nothing about the way in which the poor live; how their over-crowding destroys all sense of personal dignity, of modesty, of outer decency, till human life, as Bishop Fraser justly said, is "degraded below the level of the swine." To such and among such I went, and I could not grudge the price which seemed to be the ransom for their redemption. It meant indeed the losing of all that made life dear, but it seemed to be also the gaining for them of all that gave hope of better future. So who could hesitate, whose heart had been fired by the devotion to an ideal Humanity, inspired by the Materialism that is of love and not of hate?

Unfortunately, the ideal Humanity was raised on a false pedestal, on the belief that Man was the outcome of purely physical causes, instead of their master and creator. Related but to terrestrial existence, he was but the loftiest organism of earth, and failing to see his past and his future, how should my eyes have not been blinded to the deep lying causes of his present woe? I had brought a material cure to a disease which appeared to me to be of material origin. But how when the evil was of subtler origin, and its causes lay not in the material plane? And how if the remedy set up new causes for future evil, only drove in the symptoms of the disease while intensifying the virus hidden out of sight? That was the new problem set for solution when Theosophy unrolled the story of man, told of his origin and his destiny, and shewed the true relation between his past, his present and his future.

For what is man in the light of Theosophic truth? He is a spiritual intelligence, eternal and uncreate, treading a vast cycle of human experience, born and reborn on earth millennium after millennium, evolving slowly into the Ideal man. He is not the product of matter but is encased in matter, and the forms of matter with which he clothes himself are of his own making. For the intelligence and the will of man are creative forces (not creative ex-nihilo, but creative as is the brain of the painter), and these forces are exercised by man in every act of thought; thus he is ever creating round him thought-forms, moulding subtlest matter into shape by these energies, forms which persist as tangible realities for those who have developed the senses whereby they are cognisable. Now, when the time for rebirth into this earth-life approaches, these thought-forms pass from the mental to the astral plane, and become denser through the building into them of astral matter; and into these astral forms in turn are built the molecules of physical matter, which matter is thus moulded for the new body on the lines laid down by the intelligent and volitional life of the previous, or of many previous, incarnations. So does each man create for himself in verity the form wherein he functions, and what he is in his present is the inevitable outcome of his own creative energies in his past.

It is not difficult to see how this view of man will affect the neo-Malthusian theory. Physical man in the present being largely the result of mental man in the past, complicated by the instincts physically transmitted and arising from the deeds of the physical body, and being only the tool or medium where through the true self works on the physical plane, all that man needs to do is to keep his tool in the best working order for his highest purposes, training it in responsiveness to the impulses of the noblest that is in him. Now the sexual instinct that he has in common with the brute is one of the most fruitful sources of human misery, and the satisfaction of its imperious cravings is at the root of most of the trouble of the world. To hold this instinct in complete control to develop the intellectual at the expense of the animal (nature, and thus to raise the whole man from the animal) to the human stage, such is the task to which humanity should set itself. The excessive development of this instinct in man far greater and more constant than in any brute has to be fought against, and it will most certainly never be lessened by easy-going self-indulgence within the marital relation, any more than by self-indulgence outside it. It has reached its present abnormal development by self-indulgence in the past, all sexual thoughts, desires, and imaginations having created their appropriate thought forms, into which have been wrought the brain and body molecules which now give rise to passion on the material plane. By no other road than by that of self-control and self-denial can men and women now set going the causes which on their future return to earth life shall build for them bodies and brains of a higher type. The sooner the causes are started the sooner the results will accrue; from which it follows that Theosophists should sound the note of self-restraint within marriage, and the restriction of the marital relation to the perpetuation of the race. Such is the inevitable outcome of the Theosophic theory of man's nature, as inevitably as neo-Malthusianism was the outcome of the Materialist theory. Passing from Materialism to Theosophy, I must pass from neo-Malthusianism to what will be called asceticism, and it is right to state this clearly, since my name has been so long and so publicly associated with the other teaching. I have refused either to print any more or to sell the copyright of the "Law of Population," so that when those that have passed beyond my control have been disposed of by those who bought them, no more copies will be circulated. I only lately came to this definite decision, for I confess my heart somewhat failed me at the idea of withdrawing from the knowledge of the poor, so far as I could, a palliative of the heart-breaking misery under which they groan, and from the married mothers of my own sex, the impulse to aid whom had been my strongest motive of action in 1877, a protection against the evils which too often wreck their lives and bring many to an early grave, worn old before even middle age has touched them. Not until I felt obliged to admit that the neo-Malthusianism teaching was anti-Theosophical, would I take this step: but, having taken it, it is right to take it publicly, and to frankly say that my former teaching was based on a mistaken view of man's nature, treating him as the mere product of evolution instead of as the spirit intelligence and will without which evolution could not be.

Many will be inclined to ask: "Are you not sorry that you suffered so much for what was based on a mistaken view of human life?" Frankly, no. From that arduous and painful struggle, into which I entered against all the instincts of my nature and in defiance of my social training, from the sole desire to help the poor and the suffering, I have learned lessons which I would not have missed for the sake of any escape from pain. I learned in it to stand alone, careless of ill-informed or self seeking opinion; to face opprobrium for the sake of principle, social ostracism for the sake of duty, hatred for the sake of love. The method was mistaken, but the principle was right, and this at least is the fruit of that past bitter struggle: the strength to embrace an unpopular cause, to face ridicule and stem opposition, strength which may have its place for service in defence of that Cause to which my Leader and Teacher H. P. B. judged me worthy to dedicate my life.

# INDEX OF NAMES

# INDEX OF SUBJECTS

For Product Safety Concerns and Information please contact our EU
representative  GPSR@taylorandfrancis.com
Taylor & Francis Verlag GmbH, Kaufingerstraße 24, 80331 München, Germany